The Harry Secombe Diet Book

Robson Books

FIRST PUBLISHED IN GREAT BRITAIN IN 1983 BY
ROBSON BOOKS LTD., BOLSOVER HOUSE, 5-6
CLIPSTONE STREET, LONDON W1P 7EB. COPY-
RIGHT © 1983 SIR HARRY SECOMBE.
DIET SHEETS ON PAGES 42-73 COPYRIGHT © 1983
SLIMLINE (WEIGHT REDUCTIONS) LTD.

First impression March 1983
Second impression April 1983
Third impression April 1983
Fourth impression June 1983
Fifth impression October 1983
Sixth impression June 1984
Seventh impression April 1985
Eighth impression March 1987

Secombe, *Sir* Harry
    The Harry Secombe diet book.
    1. Reducing diets   2. Physical fitness
    I. Title
    613.2'5   RM222.2

    ISBN 0-86051-229-0
    ISBN 0-86051-230-4 Pbk

Jacket design by Harold King

Printed and bound in Great Britain by
Biddles Ltd, Guildford and King's Lynn

Contents

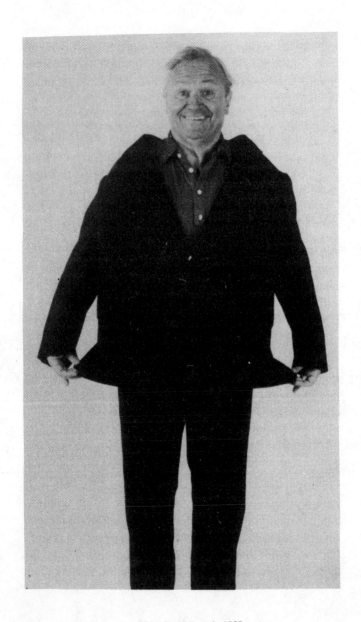

Photo David Secombe 1983

Foreword

Hands up all those who jumped up to adjust the horizontal hold on their television sets when I made my first appearance as Slimline Secombe. Yes, folks, I've done it at last. Half a hundredweight of lard has disappeared like the snow melts on the top of Tommy Cooper with the first touch of spring.

For years I have been making excuses for being fat, pretending that I liked lugging all that extra weight about; getting stuck in lifts, wedged in doorways, bursting water beds and having to get sail makers to make my shirts. But now I have burst free from my cocoon of suet and a new figure has emerged. I can see my feet again; strange xylophone-like objects have appeared at the side of my chest which, my wife informs me, are ribs. My knees and elbows blink in the unaccustomed light.

What's happened to me is not the result of a slow puncture, it is all because I have been on a diet. Not one of those crash diets where you put all the weight back on again in a few weeks, but a proper diet to which you can adhere and which you can enjoy. I am greatly indebted to Patricia Dunne-North of Slimline Weight Reductions Ltd., who first introduced my wife, Myra, to this highly efficient way of shedding the old avoirdupois. Myra adapted the Slimline diet to suit my particular needs and it is with Pat's collaboration that this book has been produced. I would also like to thank Denise Winn for her invaluable assistance and all the medical research she's done for this book.

There is no doubt about it, this is an eminently practical diet. It is easy to follow and, as you can see from the way I look now, it works. Come on, fatties, beat inflation — discover the new you underneath the old one. You've got nothing to lose but your gains.

February, 1983   H.S.

Big fat Harry

It is fitting that I should begin this book with a confession. For years I have pretended that I loved being fat. "Fat is beautiful," I would cry from the rooftops, and all the time inside my elephantine shape there was a gazelle trying to get out. Apart from the fact that I was aware of taking up too much space in an already overcrowded world, the discomfort of being over nineteen stone was beginning to tell on me. I kept thinking that I was being followed, and all the time it was me. It was getting obvious to those near and dear to me that an eclipse of the "Goon" was on the cards. Whenever I plodded my way around a golf course local seismologists registered me as scoring seven on the Richter Scale. Cyril Smith was hinting that if I had any old suits to spare he was in the market for them. Of course I didn't send him any — let's face it, they would have been too big for him.

How did it all start then, you ask. When did I start putting on the weight? Well, to begin with, I was not a fat child, in fact quite the opposite. "He looks like a fourpenny rabbit," said my Uncle Harry when he first saw me. My early childhood was marked by various colourful illnesses — scarlet fever, yellow jaundice — I only needed black-water fever to complete the spectrum.

But I was well on the road to being a fat man even when I was a kid, though I didn't realise — or care about — it then. My mother had the kind of bosom you could hurl yourself into and get lost. She was always in the kitchen, ladling out love in the form of pot roasts and pastries. After a hard day at school sharpening pencils and cleaning the blackboard I came to associate release from the grind of grammar and geometry with the mouthwatering smells wafting out of the kitchen at home. Other little boys used to wake up in the morning thinking, "Oh crumbs. Today's PE and I haven't done my algebra homework." I'd think, "Yippee! It's steak and kidney pud tonight, with lots of chips, and baked jam roll with custard for afters!"

Sunday was best. Bacon and eggs and laverbread — that's seaweed, honestly! — plenty of fried bread for breakfast, followed by a huge roast with all the trimmings for Sunday lunch and then another big fry-up that night. I didn't need a watch or a calendar, I could tell the time and day by the smells that wafted into the living room.

In spite of all this I was only ten stone six when, as a young soldier, I was sent to Italy. I soon discovered the delights of pasta. I ate spaghetti by the yard, swimming in rich creamy sauces. Then, just so as not to feel too nostalgic for home, the other boys and I would cook up crates of good old eggs and chips. So I was beginning to put on weight when I finally returned to civvy street in 1946.

Soon after demobilisation I met Myra at a dance back home in Swansea. I arranged to meet her at the Plaza cinema the next week and then, as I hadn't been wearing my glasses at the dance, I got cold feet. I decided to hide behind a pillar until she came and then make the decision whether to come out or not. Nobody turned up. After half an hour I gave it up as a bad job and emerged from behind my pillar — just as Myra was emerging from behind hers. She had had the same idea. If I had weighed as much then as I did six months ago, she'd have seen me straight off and would probably have faded away home as fast as she could scuttle. I can't imagine what life would have been like if she had. I became the man I am because of Myra — in more ways than one. I always say her gravy was my downfall. She says I only married her because she looks Italian and reminded me of my beloved spaghetti.

I was trying to make it as a professional entertainer by this time and everywhere I went my wife came with me. What a joy it was, during summer seasons in Brixham or Blackpool, to come home to some real Welsh cooking. She cooked me all my favourites, spaghetti, egg and chips, steak and kidney, with lashings of that indescribable gravy. I had developed such an obsession for potatoes by this time that I had to have mountains of them, baked, fried, roasted, mashed or boiled, for every meal. I was so worried that she wouldn't be able to peel them fast enough that I even bought her a special kind of peeling machine which only meant turning a handle.

Meanwhile poor old Myra was going potty. I had to have two cooked meals a day, so that old housewife's dilemma of "what shall I cook tonight" was daily doubled. Many was the time she would gaze at me in despair when I'd devour a whole meal of soup and steak and chips and vegetables and home-made apple pie, punctuated with slices of thick buttered bread, and then say, "Well, what's next? I'm starving!" So out would come the cheese and biscuits and fruit.

Because of my work, most nights I wouldn't get my evening meal till after the show, maybe later than twelve o'clock at night. I'd wallop it all down, three huge courses, and then stagger straight to bed. Does wonders for your digestion that does. It's all still there, sitting in your stomach, next morning, groaning at the prospect of a whole cooked breakfast slithering down to join it.

On top of all this, I had by now developed quite a taste for Guinness but that didn't last too long as I started to balloon out even more. So I acquired the taste for strange concoctions instead, like whisky and ginger ale or coke and brandy. They looked so innocent and elegant they just couldn't be fattening I thought, in my ignorant bliss. I even went through a Pernod period. "There's more water than Pernod, so that must be all right," I'd say to Myra. I introduced her to it too, by taking her to those little pavement cafés in Paris and ordering it for the pair of us. But, oh dear, it wouldn't be long before the waiters would come round with little taste-bud tempters on a tray, crates of calories compressed into little canapés.

I wasn't ever that much of a drinker but I did love milk. I'd down half a pint before going out and then, after a show, I'd walk in the door, open the fridge, and swallow a whole pint at one go. Singing is thirsty work, I'd tell myself. All Myra could do was change from Gold Top to Silver. Since I've stopped drinking it whole herds of Jerseys have become unemployed. I

8

would look ruefully at my ballooning belly and say to her, "It's all your fault. It would never have happened if it hadn't been for your gravy," and she'd open those lovely brown eyes wide and wail, "But it wasn't my fault you drank all that milk and Guinness!"

On Sundays she would yell at me the most when I'd say to the kids, "Here, run to the shop and buy a few boxes of chocolates."

When the Goons took off, I thought I had a reason to maintain my generous proportions. I was known as "the fat one", it paid me not to be thin. Years later when I played the title role in the musical *Pickwick*, there was a scene in which I had to strut around the stage in a bald wig, weaving my way in and out of the chorus whilst singing "Turkeys bigger than I am . . .". My mind used to seize up at the thought of poultry weighing over 17 stone. I imagined the struggle to get it into the oven . . . cold turkey sandwiches continuing well into July.

Not that it stopped me. Many was the time after three good meals in a day that Myra and I would lie in bed and I would say in a tiny voice, "Myra, I've got the *gwilda*." That's our Welsh expression for the hollow feeling that hits the stomach at night. And one or both of us would end up downstairs in the kitchen, having a midnight feast of tea and toast. Even the tea would have five spoonfuls of sugar in it.

When I hit it big in my career at last, I also hit it big on my belly. There was a whole new world out there — and it all had food in it. If I was working abroad, I had to fly and that meant whiling away the airborne hours with all the drinks and juices and snacks and meals they cared to wheel in my direction. I had to have a special extension put on my seatbelt, though there was little risk of my being hurled out of my seat in a touch of turbulence. On the contrary, when we landed, I had to wait till the other passengers had got off before someone had time to come and lever me out.

I've worked in Australia a lot and I love it, though I'm afraid Australian hospitality is overwhelming — especially where cans of lager are concerned. But Majorca was the place where I really had the chance to indulge in my love of red wine. When Myra and I bought ourselves a home there, it would be red wine with lunch and red wine with dinner, to say nothing of an aperitif by the pool. And the food! Everything that could be fried in batter

9

was fried in batter and topped with a ton of oil. Lovely. And lethal. But I didn't care.

"Go on," I'd say to Myra, "*that* won't hurt you," as I ladled pasta or fried and stuffed peppers on to her plate. Salad or chips, what difference did it make which one you chose, as long as you only chose one, if you were trying to diet. (It was Myra who was always trying to diet, not me. I wouldn't have known a calorie if it had hit me in the face. Unfortunately it used to hit me in the stomach.)

"Well, at least you don't eat *between* meals," Myra would say, grateful for minuscule mercies. "But that is because life is one long meal," I'd joke. "There isn't any time in-between."

In 1979 I had to have major surgery for an abscess on the colon which had burst. I lost two stone through illness and learned that I was diabetic to boot. That was a shock and I laid off all the sugary stuff, but it didn't stop me eating. Three years later I was back to 19 stone. Myra was pleading with me to lose weight, to try one of her diets, to cut down if not out, but I wasn't having any of it. It was too much effort and, besides, I thought, I felt fine. I was fit. I could sing. Even if I couldn't walk without wheezing, and getting out of an armchair required as much effort as twenty press-ups and a backward roll.

Then came the fateful interview with a blunt Australian doctor. I was singing at the Sydney Opera House and felt in imminent danger of collapse. After the show I found myself stripped to the buff being examined by a no-messing-around doctor from Woolloomoolloo. His own blood pressure went up when he took mine and that was before he even got to my blood sugar. He looked at me straight and said, "Keep this up and I give you two years at the most."

My heart turned over and I felt so ill I believed him. I was 61 and had lots left in me — or could have. Then my terror turned to anger — with myself. I was being utterly selfish the way I lived my life. I had a wonderful wife and four wonderful children and I was going to ruin life for them if I carried on ruining my own. I made up my mind there and then that I was going to change my lifestyle. I'm now a five stones lighter and happier man and I know, without a quaver of doubt, that big fat Harry will never be seen again.

I'm going to tell you how I did it so that you can do it too.

Time for a shock

Okay, I had an incentive to lose weight — and fast. I was given a short sharp shock by a very direct doctor and it finally hit home. This is it, Harry boy, I said to myself. You either give up your lifestyle or you give up your life. No other choice. I realised for the first time how I had abused my body right through my life, not just by filling it up with fat but by making impossible demands of it. Like thinking "the show must go on", even when I had a broken arm or pneumonia, Martyrdom? It was madness. And Myra always told me so.

But all Myra's loving concern, all her efforts and urgings, didn't have the power to make me change my ways, though God knows I think the world of her. I knew she would love me whatever I was like. I knew she would still fancy me even if I looked like an elephant. And that is why love can't do what fear can. Only a doctor's dire prognosis could snap me out of my Harry-go-lucky ways. *He* told me my luck had run out.

If you are overweight and wish you weren't, you need a shock like I had to get you moving. But you don't need to wait till it gets so late. Because I am going to give you your shock now.

You know if you are really fat or not. And if you are, everything — but everything — I am going to say now applies to *you.*

The Royal College of Physicians recently produced a report on obesity. They were alarmed to find that 30 per cent of adults and five per cent of children are too fat for their own good.

Nearly eight per cent are actually obese — that means weighing 20 per cent more than the recommended upper weight limit for your height and frame. We are unhealthy eaters and are suffering the consequences of it, says the College. Here's why.

Despite what we think of our economy we live in a rich country when it comes to food. The richer the country, the richer the food. So we eat more sugar, more eggs, more fats, more milk, more meat than people in poorer countries. And we eat less of cereals, fruit and vegetables. Now let us compare health. In rich countries we suffer much more heart disease, obesity, diabetes, cancer, tooth decay and mental stress. In poor countries the killers are infectious diseases — and starvation. Not all our illnesses can be laid at the door of what we eat and how much. But a lot can. Look at the list.

Overweight and heart disease

Heart disease is the cause of death for 30 per cent of people. It is the biggest killer of all. If you are fat, you are twice as likely to be at risk. If you smoke and have high blood pressure as well, your chances of escaping it are even slimmer — especially if the disease runs in your family anyway. Men are more susceptible than women, but women once over 60 are at almost equal risk.

It might be coincidence that people in countries that eat most fat have the highest rates for heart disease. But there definitely seems to be a link between the amount and type of fat you eat and the fatty deposits that build up in the arteries. The heart needs a constant flow of oxygen to do its work and if fatty deposits build up in the arteries (called the 'coronary arteries') that supply the heart muscle, not enough oxygen gets through. This, especially when the heart is beating faster because of stress or exercise, leads to the constricting pain of angina that spreads across the chest. If the arteries to the heart become too narrow, the blood may clot causing a coronary heart attack. Even if you don't eat a tremendous amount of fat but you are still overweight, just carrying that load around with you is enough to put strain on your heart.

Overweight and high blood pressure

Doctors now believe that being too fat contributes directly to high blood pressure. Slim people are far less likely to get it. If you have really high blood pressure, you are at greater risk of having a heart problem or even a stroke.

If you have high blood pressure, it means that the blood is being pumped through your arteries with a great force and this can lead to strain on the arteries as well. You may not know that you have high blood pressure because it is usually symptomless. Only in rare or extremely severe cases are there signs such as headaches, fluttery feelings or general ill health, though it must be stressed that people can have these symptoms without a high blood pressure. Don't think you'll go red in the face or sweat a lot if you have anything to worry about from high blood pressure. Those are myths.

But it isn't a myth that you put far too much strain on your circulatory system of you are overweight and that is when the troubles can start.

Men are at risk more than women and the risk increases as you become older.

Overweight and stroke

Though many with a stroke may suffer no *permanent* damage, sometimes this is not the case. A stroke is caused by the same sort of problem that leads to high blood pressure and heart attacks. The arteries get clogged, usually with fatty deposits, and blood can't flow through easily. In the case of stroke, however, it is one of the arteries supplying the brain that gets blocked and the brain can't function properly. Let us help to keep our brains functioning properly by not overeating!

Overweight and diabetes

Diabetes mellitus is a disease you can get when the pancreas has problems making insulin. In middle-aged adults it is associated with being overweight. When people have diabetes, they have an excess of glucose in their blood, and their own bodies can't produce enough insulin to deal with it. The result is high blood sugar. The excess sugar spills into the urine, which sometimes makes you need to urinate frequently and to feel extreme thirst and fatigue.

Seventy-five per cent of all adults with diabetes are overweight. They have a higher risk of hardening of the arteries, and uncontrolled diabetes can also lead to many other complications.

Overweight and diverticulitis

Diverticulitis, from which I suffer, is not helped by a bad diet, and as most overweight people tend to eat a lot of the wrong foods, some may come to suffer this complaint. Diverticulitis is an inflammation in the swelling of the small pouches that sometimes develop on the walls of the colon. When people eat the wrong foods — too much egg and milk and cheese and meat which don't have any roughage — the muscles of the colon get overstrained and weak spots, like pouches, may form in certain susceptible people. Bits of waste material may get trapped there and become impacted. The inflammation can develop. An acute attack can cause severe pain, and may be difficult to clear up — antibiotic treatment may be necessary. To prevent further attacks, or indeed an initial one, a correct diet, containing plenty of fibre (what we used to call 'roughage' — there's more about it on page 32) is strongly recommended.

Overweight and constipation

Constipation is also caused by eating too much of the wrong foods and putting too much strain on the veins under the lining of the rectum and the anus. The body finds it difficult to deal with refined foods, like cakes and chocolates and white bread, especially in excess and untempered by fibrous foods, such as cereals and fruits and vegetables. As constipation leads to straining, the veins around the anus become swollen and twisted and easily get ruptured.

14

Overweight and tooth decay

Fewer than 30 per cent of people ever go to a dentist for check-ups. A great many of those who don't will lose all their teeth. Decay is caused by eating sugar and most fat people eat far more in sugar than people who are slim. Fat people are also the more likely to get up in the middle of the night for a snack, perhaps a sugary one, after they have cleaned their teeth. Sugar left on the teeth is then worked on by bacteria and forms plaque. The bacteria breaks down the sugar and makes acid which eats away at the tooth enamel and makes a tiny hole — that gets bigger and bigger.

Overweight and gallstones

The gallbladder stores bile which is a fluid that is released after meals to help in the digestion of fats. A gallstone is a small solid particle which collects in the gallbladder and then grows as more fatty material hardens round it. Gallstones are found far more commonly in people who have high levels of fat in their blood and most commonly in people who are considerably overweight. Some gallstones don't produce symptoms but others get stuck in the bile duct and cause intense pain and sometimes nausea. Feelings of discomfort are worse after a fatty meal. If inflammation occurs, hospital treatment will probably be necessary.

Overweight and varicose veins

If you are very fat you are especially prone to suffer varicose veins. About one person in a hundred gets them and women are three times more likely to have them than men. Varicose veins are twisted, swollen veins and they can often be unsightly. They occur when blood is squeezed the wrong way and veins have to swell and twist to hold it. They usually occur in the legs, look bluish and can be tender and itchy. Sometimes they make the whole leg ache and the feet seem to swell. At best they are uncomfortable. At worst they can cause ulcers or require surgery.

Overweight and arthritis

You don't just put extra strain on your heart if you are fat. You put extra strain on your joints and ligaments which have to move your bulk around. That can often put you at higher risk of arthritis. Arthritis usually hits the weight-bearing joints — the knees, hips or spine. The bones, where they touch each other around the cartilage, start to flake because of overuse. The cartilage starts to waste away and the bone becomes heavy and swollen. Movement becomes painful and sometimes there is a flare-up of inflammation. It isn't dangerous but it can be miserable and can mean a change in lifestyle, if the pain is severe enough to interfere with your everyday life.

Whether fat people fall prey to arthritis or not, because they are so large they have trouble moving quickly and often their balance is poor. This tends to mean that they are far more likely to have accidents at home or at work.

Overweight and hospital hazards

When very fat people need surgery, perhaps for a disease totally unconnected with their weight, their fat may present more of a problem to the surgeon and the anaesthetist. The eminent surgeon Dickson Wright once said that if he ever had to operate on me he would "wear a bikini and a pair of wellingtons, use a six-foot scalpel and stand well back". Too much bodyweight can make general anaesthetic more of a risk. A grossly overweight woman may also have extreme difficulty giving birth.

Overweight and depression

Fat people are supposed to be jolly but a great many spend a lot of time feeling depressed. They don't think they look good, therefore they start not to *feel* good. They yearn to fit into fashionable clothes, to enjoy a meal without thinking of their waistline, to be able to join in sports or dance or do all the fun things slim people do without even thinking. They fear they are not attractive to the opposite sex, and they can end up with a very poor self-image.

Those, then, are the facts and I have put them brutally bluntly because I know what a power of good plain speaking can do. I only wish someone had said it to me much earlier. So now I hope you really do want to lose weight as much as I did. The next step is to break that fatal habit of "thinking fat".

Stop rationalising

I made part of my career out of being fat. My act would be peppered with "fat" jokes — "I was 6ft 3in when I was twelve but I was hit by a lift"; "I have to be a middle of the road singer — there's no room for me on the pavement"; "I'm an all *round* entertainer" — and so on. I had some diet jokes too. "Outside every fat man there's a thin man screaming to get in", and my diet tip used to be "Eat as much as you like but don't swallow." Spike Milligan always referred to me as "that well-known danger to shipping" and "my favourite singing group".

I felt affectionate towards my fat — or I told myself I did. When I was all dolled up in an evening suit, I'd pat my enormous belly and say, "pot black". Everybody laughed and I laughed with them. You see, I never really accepted that I was fat. That sounds ridiculous, a nineteen-stone mountain not thinking he was fat. But I didn't. Or rather, I didn't think I was *too* fat. That's the first illusion that has got to go if you want to diet. Look at yourself and face it: "I'm much too fat." Stop saying, "Well, if I turn slightly sideways" or "That mirror always was a bit wonky." It isn't true and you know it.

Now let's get rid of the rest of those rationalisations we all like to resort to.

Fat people are jolly

That's what I used to say. Even fat words sounded much more friendly and comforting than thin ones. I would savour the

18

sound of words like fat, jolly, jumbo, plump, chubby, and fat-associated words like butter, lard and balloon. Whereas I would dismiss as sinister words like lean, gaunt, thin, skinny, bony and angular. Being fat meant cuddly, jolly and comforting. But when I was saying those things, even though I was a happy fat man, deep down I secretly wished I was slim. Next time you try kidding yourself, remember how often you've wept into the fish and chips.

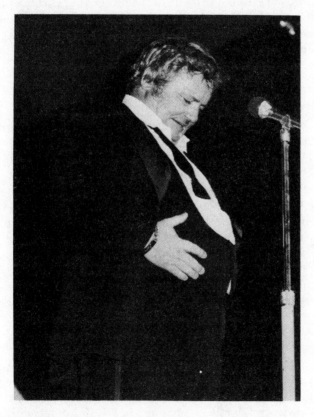

Pot black, 1980

People love me as I am

Yes, people love you as you are — and they'll love you whatever you are, if they really care for you. I've said it before, Myra never stopped loving me even when I was a ton of lard. But she hasn't stopped loving me now either, now that I'm a stripling instead of a thundering great oak. If you fear you will lose your friends or lover if you slim down to the real you, either you have too low an opinion of yourself or they don't love the real you at all. It isn't so unknown, unfortunately, for more slender acquaintances of your own sex to encourage your excesses just so that they can be sure to be the centre of attraction when you are together. But think carefully. Is it really they who are stopping you slimming or you who is stopping yourself by using them?

I get heartburn but it's stress

That was another of my old favourites. After tucking into a three course meal and demolishing a loaf of bread between courses, I'd coolly blame my heartburn on overwork. "That's what does it," I'd say to Myra, as I painfully subsided into the only armchair large enough, "I'm working too hard, what with all these rehearsals for concerts and TV shows." And she would give me one of those looks that I didn't see. When you are kidding yourself, you can't afford to look. So next time you catch yourself saying, "It's standing up so much that makes me tired" or "Of course, at my age you can't expect . . ." just remember — it's rubbish and you know it. I know it. I don't have heartburn any more — but the stress is still there.

It's vain to look in mirrors anyway

Who cares if it *is* vain to look in mirrors. It's fun — if you've got something nice to see. I can't keep away from mirrors now — it is so long since I dared look in one I nearly didn't recognise my face, let alone my body. The only reason people don't look in mirrors is if they don't want to face the awful fact — they're fat. As if it will go away if they don't have to look at it. Defiant shakes of the head and protestations of "I don't care what I look like" don't deceive anyone, least of all yourself. We all want to look attractive, whatever it is that attractive means to us. The one thing it doesn't mean to anyone is mountains of blubber spilling over shoes and cuffs and waistbands in rubbery rolls.

Knowing my luck . . .

Knowing my luck, I'll spend three months dieting religiously, eating nothing but cottage cheese and lettuce and being miserable, and then, the very day that I'm a svelte new me, I'll step out in front of a bus. That was one of my old favourites too. It's really a recipe for not doing anything in life at all. After all, why bother to undergo the fag of learning to drive or learning a trade or getting out of bed. That bus could always be lurking round the corner. Funny really, considering there seem to be so few around when you want them.

Who wants to live long anyway?

Popular line with fat people and smokers. Who wants to be elderly and have arthritis and various diseases and not to be able to get around like you used to? Why not enjoy life now and let it be short but fun? Of course it doesn't work like that. If you are overweight, your life certainly might be shorter than it ought to be. But, short as it is, it probably won't be a healthy or a fun one. You read the list in the previous chapter? All that lot could be yours well before you are drawing your old age pension. All that lot will probably be yours even if you don't get as far as drawing your old age pension. Don't kid yourself you'll be fit to the finish, then pop like a balloon.

I won't be me any more

Well, you can't kid *me* with that one, even if you can kid yourself. I wasn't just fat Harry to my family and friends, I was fat Harry right across the world. I really did use to think that if

I wasn't fat, I'd be so much not me, I'd be out of a job. And I had five mouths to feed even if mine didn't need it. Now I'm not fat and I'm still the same old me. So I'm not a funny fat man, I'm a funny thinner man. Because I haven't lost my sense of humour, I've still got my laugh, I can still hit a top "C" and blow raspberries with the best of them. In fact, it is only now I am thinner that I can truly see how little my personality was tied up with my weight. I think I'd be jolly even if I was skinny — although I'm not going that far. If I was making it for the first time as a Goon now, I wouldn't be the fat one, I'd be the something else one. Don't ask me what, but someone would have thought of something. They always do.

I'm unhappy when I'm thin

A dubious one that, as few of us fatties have ever been thin long enough to know. But if it is really true, it is because you may have lost weight but you still thought fat. You thought of all the things you believed were lost instead of all the things you gained. You didn't take advantage of your new freedom from fat to do all sorts of things that you yearned to do when fat. You probably just sat about yearning for the things you couldn't do when thin. And there's only one. Eat. Maybe you even thought you must be different as a person if you were thin instead of realising that the essential you is always the same. If you had difficulty recognising yourself and being comfortable with yourself, perhaps it was because you too were duped by those layers of fat into thinking they made up the real you. Perhaps you were unhappy because you could no longer hide behind your fat and because people suddenly started to notice and admire you. You couldn't handle it because secretly you were thinking fat and that no one could admire *you*. Don't give in and bolt for the biscuits. Face the facts, conquer the old fears — and enjoy it.

It's just puppy fat

That might be true if you are in your teens. Changes in the sex hormones in your body during adolescence can add on a bit of body fat, especially for girls. But if you overeat as well — and you know if you do — you'll get the kind of fat that has nothing to do with puppies. It won't drop off like magic at 21. And if you are over 21 and still talking about puppy fat — stop kidding yourself. Your fat is there to stay unless you do something about it.

It's my metabolism

It is true that different people's metabolisms work at different rates. Two people of different body types can eat exactly the same diet and while one puts on the pounds the other stays lean and lithe. But even if you are one of the unlucky ones, that is generally no excuse for giving up and shovelling in the cakes and cream. You can usually lose weight, it just means you have to work harder at it for longer. All the more reason to forget the delights of over-indulgence and re-educate your appetite for life.

It's my glands

It usually isn't. Very few people have a glandular problem that accounts for their overweight.

It's in my genes

After all, it must be. My mother's fat, my father's fat, my sister's fat ... Nice try, but even the experts are now looking askance at that one. Probably your family *is* fat because you've all been encouraged to overeat. My mother certainly encouraged me, although with the best intentions in the world. If you learn at home as a child to eat and enjoy big meals, you are likely to carry on doing it as an adult — and to teach your own children to do it as well. It isn't a genetic trait, it is just a habit, in most cases. Some people, sadly, do inherit a tendency towards fat and it affects the metabolism. As said above, it just means working harder to beat the flab.

I look all right – don't I?

Fat people will do anything not to see the truth. I can remember the feeling when I used to get out my cricket gear for my once-yearly charity match. That's funny, I'd think, struggling into my whites. They've spent a year sitting doing nothing in my bag and now they seem to have shrunk. My cricket bag must have developed some mysterious shrinking propensities during that time.

Fat people will do anything but face the awful glaring reality of why the waistband doesn't meet. We'll squeeze ourselves into our clothes, now two sizes too small, ignore the sound of seams parting company and buttons bouncing on to the floor, and sigh with relief. We've got it on at last, so it must be all right.

Christmas is coming up

Christmas is always coming up. So is lunch with the relations and the birthday dinner at the special Italian retaurant. There is always a reason not to start a diet. Another good one is stress. When you've enough to cope with, whether it's keeping three vocal children under five out of mischief, taking on a new job or studying for exams, the last thing you want to have to think of on top is not eating. Not eating takes a lot of thought. Much better to wait till you have time to spare and haven't a million other inconvenient things to take your mind off it. Fortunately that time never comes, so you don't have to diet.

I'll start tomorrow

That means "I can justify having five helpings of chips and a cream puff pastry today". Starting tomorrow never means anything if you only thought of it yesterday. It's a private con designed to take away, temporarily, the guilt of over-indulging. If you are really going to start tomorrow, you have to psych yourself into it and get yourself into a dieting frame of mind. That does not come easily while cramming down the crusty rolls.

It's rude to say no . . .

How can I possibly refuse Aunty Muriel's Welsh cakes, she'll be so upset? You want to know how? Tell her, before you visit, that you are on a diet and you really don't want her to tempt you. But you can only do that if you really mean it, of course. When you are having dinner in someone else's house, you *can* watch the portions and ask for a small one. You *can* leave some food on your plate. You will if you really want to. But I know how it feels to be so trapped by courtesy on some occasions that you just have to say yes to a little treat when you really want to say no. Myra and I, while on holiday, were begged to visit an old friend and she had spent the entire morning making cakes. I just had to have a tiny slice of Madeira. Funny thing was that I was so determined to diet that I really didn't want it. When I ate it I felt terrible, like a cheat. But the important thing was that I took it in my stride. I didn't throw in the towel and attack the rest of the tea trolley. I couldn't have stayed firm if I hadn't felt confident and committed to my pledge to lose weight.

I'll do the apple diet, it always works

Apple diet, water diet, chips diet, cheese diet, they all promise to lose you pounds and stones in about three days flat. How can they work if you are back to the size you are? They are just an insurance policy, but not a health one, that allows you to pack in the pie and pastry beforehand. "It'll be all right, it will all come off on my magic fat-melting desperation diet!" You know it doesn't work for long enough to make much dent. It is the equivalent of the old smokers' joke. "Giving up smoking is easy. I've done it hundreds of times."

I don't eat anything

And yet I put on all this weight. The familiar wail of fatties everywhere. Sometimes it is true, if you are unlucky enough to have a slow metabolism. But most of the time we eat more than we think. A little won't hurt, we say. But a little soon becomes a lot if it is a biscuit snatched several times a day or just an eensy-weensy bit of butter on numerous slices of bread. Have you ever tried keeping an eaters' diary, noting down every single morsel that passes your lips in a day? It can give you quite a shock when you count up the calories.

But it's such a comfort

Oh yes, it can be such a comfort all right, when you are feeling bored or lonely or depressed. Just a little bit of yesterday's apple pie or a nice bar of chocolate makes all the difference — for the ten seconds it takes to eat it. And then what are you going to do for comfort for the rest of the evening? Feel guilt and self-loathing straight away (do you ever eat comfort food *without* feeling bad after?) or put off the evil moment a bit longer by raiding the larder and devouring all and everything first? At least you won't be bored or lonely any more. You'll be too busy being guilty and hating yourself to have time for that.

I'll go to a sauna

I can't face dieting but if I go to a sauna instead I'll lose pounds without any effort. Wrong and you know it. The miraculous drop of the needle on the scales is registering the amount of fluid you have lost in sweat. You can sit and wallow and perspire like a piglet but it will all go back on the minute you drink your first glass of water. Would that we could sweat fat — but we can't. You know it, I know it, there's no cutting corners or easy ways when it comes to losing weight. Appetite suppressants, pills that purport to make you feel full, they are all just ways of putting off the crucial moment — the day you start to diet.

It isn't masculine to diet

Isn't it? If anyone said I was a sissy because I'd lost weight, I'd punch him on the nose. But some men do think it isn't quite macho to be crunching on a carrot and toying with a lettuce leaf.

Well, all I can say is it isn't quite macho to be fat. I think of myself in the old days on the beach. Instead of preening myself proudly, I'd be lying there like a stranded whale, all bluster and blubber. You can swagger along the sand much better without a big pink hummock in front. I really do think, though, we've passed the time when slimming was the prerogative only of women. Men are much more conscious of their health and looks these days. If you find yourself at a party drinking mineral water or slim-line tonic, you'll probably notice others doing it too.

Men like a woman to be cuddly

You can be cuddly without being so fat that you smother the would-be cuddler. There's something faintly frightening about being swallowed up in folds of flesh, my slimmer male friends tell me. Cuddliness is about something other than being a cushion. It is the way you express warmth and the way you hold people and allow yourself to be held. Cuddliness comes from the inside out. You *can* be slim and cuddly.

It's unhealthy to be too thin

So who is asking you to be a skinny rake? It is as unhealthy to be obsessed about being thin as it is to be reluctant to let go of fat. But there is a middle course and that's what I for one am aiming at. When I was fat I used to think the only alternative was being thin and as that was so remote a possibility as to be out of the question, I was able to abandon all my flimsy fancies of reform. But there is an in-between state and it's called being right for your frame and height. It's called being the weight at which you feel truly comfortable. And I don't mean comfortable if you are safely off your feet in a supported supine position; I mean comfortable when you are running for a bus.

Life won't be worth living if I can't eat what I like

It is. I can assure you.

What you need to know about food

Six months ago, as far as I was concerned, a calorie was just one of those abstract things that made you put on weight. I've had a lot to learn about energy requirements, good foods and bad foods and what they have in them that makes them good or bad. So let's talk about what our bodies — all bodies — need to be healthy and fit before we talk about slimming diets. And explode some myths en route.

There are roughly seven things, called nutrients, our bodies need from our food: protein; fats; carbohydrates; vitamins; minerals; fibre; and water. Some of these give us our energy, which is measured in terms of our old favourite, the calorie. Calories aren't the arch-enemy, synonymous with fat and flesh. We need them to make our bodies do what we want them to. Even restful activities, like sleeping or watching TV, require energy — although not much, compared with climbing Mount Everest. If we ate the kinds of foods that gave us just as much energy as we needed to use each day, we wouldn't be putting on weight. Alas, if we eat more than we need to do whatever we are doing, our bodies store the extra up as fat.

Everybody's energy needs are different and you really need to assess your own by trial and error. It's easy enough. After a week of your normal eating pattern and your normal activity pattern, do you grow — sideways — or don't you? As a rough guide, a reasonably active woman will need about 2100 calories a day and a man between 2500 and 3000. To lose just one pound of excess flab, you need to cut from somewhere about 3500 calories. That's more than one whole day's eating. So you can see, to diet sensibly you can't think of weight loss as a short-term process, something to be done in three days flat and then abandoned in favour of your old over-eating habits. You need a sensible eating plan that gives you your energy needs without giving you extra — the basis of the diet plan in the next chapter.

Just so that that diet plan will make perfect sense, let's look at all those nutrients I mentioned earlier and see what they do to our bodies.

Protein

Proteins are essential for building and repairing body tissues. They make up an important part of our livers, brains, muscles, teeth, blood and hair, as well as of the numerous enzymes in our bodies, the substances that busy about helping us digest food. As all our cells are renewing themselves constantly, old proteins get broken down and released as energy while the body makes use of new ones.

Proteins are often referred to as amino acids because that is what they are made from. Some amino acids are formed in our bodies without any help from us but eight particular types have to be acquired through foods. We can get them in two ways, from animal and from vegetable foods. Animal proteins (from meat, fish, eggs and cheese) are very similar to our own whereas vegetable proteins have some essential bits missing, so far as our bodies are concerned. That gave rise to the old myth that vegetable proteins were therefore insufficient and if you were a vegetarian, you would waste away. In fact, if you *mix* vegetables, by eating pulses, cereals and ordinary vegetables, you get all the protein you need in a form you can use.

Let's get rid of another myth while we are at it. It isn't true that the more protein you eat, the healthier you will be, and that protein isn't fattening. No one's normal diet is likely to be low in protein because we don't need that much. But if we do eat too much, the body can't use it except as energy — or to store as fat.

Fats

We need fats for energy and also some for building and repairing parts of our bodies. They make food more tasty, as we all unfortunately know, and when we eat too much of them they get stored straight away as fat.

It is a myth that one fat is pretty much like another, although it may be that way from the weight point of view. But fats are of very different types and have different effects on the body.

Fats are either saturated or unsaturated and the first variety is believed to lead to an increase of cholesterol in the blood. We need cholesterol, a fat-like substance that plays a part in getting our hormones to function, but if we have too much, fatty deposits of the stuff start to block the arteries.

The animal fats — like that in milk, cheese, butter, eggs and meat — are thought by many authorities to be the guilty culprits when it comes to cholesterol. The vegetable fats are usually unsaturated — corn oil, soya-bean oil, sunflower and safflower oil, for instance. But beware palm and coconut oil — they are in the saturated group.

There is still some argument among the experts about whether hard fats, the animal fats, are really as bad as they have now been made out to be. But we don't have to concern ourselves with that. Because, from our point of view, as would-be slimmers, fats in any form need to be cut right down. We all eat far too much for our own good and fat-containing foods have double the calories of protein or carbohydrate-based foods.

Don't cut out fat altogether, though. We need a little of both types in our bodies.

Carbohydrates

Here's a much maligned nutrient that has had too much of a bad press for too long. You need to get it out of your head, if it is still in there, that carbohydrates, such as in bread, cereals and potatoes, are "stodge" and producers of instant inches on the waistline. Carbohydrate foods, weight for weight, have half the calories of fats. Unrefined carbohydrates (that is, wholemeal bread, flour, pasta, and so forth) are an excellent source of fibre.

There is one baddie in the carbohydrate camp, however, and that is sugar. The other types mentioned above are starches and they are useful to our bodies. Sugar, however, as bought in bags and eaten in cakes and chocolates and puddings and pies, has *no nutritional value whatsoever*. It gives us energy, sure — but so does every other food you eat.

Vitamins

Vitamins are vital for our health but we can't make them. We have to take them in in food — and they don't have any calorie value. There is a whole range of vitamins, all responsible for different things, such as good vision, good teeth, brain function, tissue repair and healing.

No one should be lacking in the right vitamins in the West if they eat the right diet. A small amount of meat, fish or dairy products, a lot of fruit and vegetables and also wholemeal bread or other grains should see you right.

Some scientists now believe that certain vitamins, particularly C and A, play an important part in helping the body to fight disease. So if you eat a lot of fruit and vegetables, where these vitamins are commonly found, you may be helping yourself to extra fitness.

You should be able to get all the vitamins from your food, without having to resort to supplements.

Minerals

We wouldn't relish the idea of eating metal if we were told to. But, in fact, we all do eat it, in minute quantities, and it is essential to our health. The minerals we need are metals and salts, such as iron, phosphorus, potassium, calcium and sodium chloride (table salt). They are all calorie-free too. They do important things like repair tissues, make teeth and bones strong, help muscles work and blood to flow and so on. Again, some scientists think they could be more important than we realise in disease-fighting. They are found in meat and vegetables and no one in this country should be deficient.

Fibre

Fibre is what used to be called roughage. It is the stuff that has revolutionalised the lives of constipation sufferers everywhere. It comes from plant sources (wholemeal grains, cereals, fruits and vegetables and pulses are high in fibre) and can't be digested by our bodies. But that doesn't mean it doesn't do us any good. Far from it. If there is a good amount of roughage passing along the intestines with all of the rest of our food waste, it will all come out the other end much quicker. By reducing pressure on the poor old colon muscles, struggling to shift wodges of fatty or stodgy foods, it makes you less at risk of diverticulitis. You should never need to take laxatives if you eat enough fibre.

Water

We mustn't forget this final calorie-free essential. We are all over two-thirds water and it is just as well, because it has a lot of work to do. All the processes in our bodies require water to work, which is why we feel so awful if we are dehydrated in any way.

Here is the good news. Many of the foods we eat, or should eat, are high in water as well. A normal person should get his or her water requirements from fluids *and* from food. Water has no calories but it is bulky, so water-high foods fill us up. Water-high foods, with the exception of things like milk which are fatty as well, are usually low in calories. It is believed that a lot of people are so overweight because they eat foods that have little water. Just chew on this: tomatoes are 93 per cent water, roast chicken is 68 per cent water, bread is 40 per cent water — and chocolate and biscuits are less than 5 per cent water.

So those are our needs. How do we translate all that into healthy eating? Here is an easy run-down of do's and don'ts.

Meat/fish

It is no bad thing to eat meat and fish, unless you are a

vegetarian, of course. But some types of each are less fattening than others. Chicken is a good low-calorie meal — if you don't eat the skin. Under the skin all that ferocious fat is hiding. Liver and kidneys are excellent meats, not only low in calories but packed with goodness. Remove all excess fat before cooking meat and always try to grill instead of fry.

Fish is excellent value as well and we tend to eat too little of it. The best for your waistline are the white varieties — cod, haddock, whiting, etc. Mackerel and tuna are high in oil — and calories.

Dairy foods

This is where life gets dangerous. Cream, milk, butter, cheese — they are all packed with fat — of the hard, less healthy, kind. You will be doing yourself a favour if you change to skimmed milk — the fat has been creamed off. And cut down your intake of hard cheeses. Edam is the lowest-calorie hard cheese and soft cheeses, such as Brie, are less fattening than good old Cheshire and Cheddar. If you can live without butter, there are plenty of vegetable oil spreads that are half the calories.

Fruit

Marvellous for you. Get into the habit of snacking on fruit instead of fudge and you are well on the way to a slimmer-line figure. All fruits are packed with goodness in the form of vitamins and minerals and, in many cases, fibre. Some are higher calorie than others, of course, but that is only relatively speaking. A good size banana is lower in calories than a tiny three-quarters of an ounce square of hard cheese.

Vegetables

Again, the things to feast on. You just couldn't tuck in enough cauliflower or broccoli to add up to the calories in two ounces of cheese. They are packed with vitamins and minerals and mostly high in fibre. Root vegetables like potatoes and parsnips are more fattening than the others but that again is relatively speaking. A filling eight-ounce potato is equivalent to our two ounces of cheese.

The experts say watch how you cook your vegetables, however, or you will be at risk of losing all the vitamins before they get near you. Don't boil too long in too much water — or else use the water as a base for soup. Don't cut up vegetables and leave them exposed to the air for too long before you use them. And never put sodium bicarbonate in the cooking water to bring out the colour of the greens. It simply destroys the vitamins.

Grains and pulses

Wholemeal bread is often lower in calories than white bread. It is much more filling and richer in fibre. The same goes for wholemeal flour and nowadays you can buy wholemeal pasta as well. Cereals, as long as they aren't loaded with sugar, are good for your body — but watch the calories. Peas, lentils and the whole range of beans are another excellent, if neglected, source of goodness. (For the 16-week diet, use the bread specified.)

Sugar

A no-no. You don't need it, your body doesn't want it and your teeth hate it. We get all the sugar we need in the form of starchy carbohydrates and fruit. It is a different kind of sugar from the kind you get in big pound bags and in cakes and chocolate. Scientists have shown that the more sugar you eat, the more food you want. They have discovered that the body signals us to stop eating when we're full by keeping tabs on the amount of glucose in the blood. But that particular thermostat only works, it seems, if the glucose enters the body slowly. When we eat sugar, it enters in a rush. The body misses the signal and allows us to carry on feeling hungry — and eating.

Your best bet is to cut out sugar — completely.

Salt

Salt doesn't put the inches on you but it is bad for you in excess in other ways. Doctors generally believe it is linked with high blood pressure. As fatties are more at risk of high blood pressure anyway, the last thing you want to do is compound the problem by eating too much salt. The experts say that we take in enough salt in food *without having to add any at the table.* So put the salt shaker at the back of the kitchen cupboard. If you find vegetables lack taste without salt, try cooking them less. You may be boiling them to pulp which makes them lose all their natural delicious flavour. But if you really really can't face some foods without salt, use a sodium-free salt such as Selora.

Alcohol

It is so easy to forget that alcohol is fattening because it doesn't feel like food. But there is a pile of calories hiding in beer — and whisky and wine and anything you care to name. The safest drink on this diet is a small whisky diluted with three times as much water (whisky, 25 per cent; water, 75 per cent). People often believe alcohol is all right on a diet because it isn't stored as fat. That is true. However, that just means that the alcohol will be used by you for energy and foods which would have been used up as energy all get stored instead around your midriff.

Supermarket foods

Convenience foods can be so appealing. Just three minutes boiling in a bag or a splash of water and you've a meal all ready to eat. But watch it when you are in supermarkets. Those tempting tins and packets all contain hidden extras — sugar and salt. Even innocent-looking tins of vegetables can have plenty of both, because sugar and salt are natural preservatives. So read labels when you buy. Some manufacturers don't put sugar in tinned vegetables. Some no longer add sugar to jam. If you are a careful shopper, you can cut down on calories you didn't even realise you were eating. And if you can't find a tin of your own particular favourite that isn't sunk in sugar and salt, leave it on the shelf.

Health food shops

Don't fall into the easy trap of thinking that health food shops must sell healthy foods. Natural sugar is no less fattening or bad for your teeth than any other sugar. Fruit bars sweetened with honey are no less likely to pack on the pounds than ordinary sugary bars. Health food shops are a good source of beans and grains, although many supermarkets now carry a fair supply. But when you are there, read the labels on the more tempting items carefully.

Those are all the rules that I've had to learn and that I'm going to stick to for life. They are ground rules for healthy eating, regardless of whether you need to lose weight or not, and they are rules we would all do well to bring up our children by.

The diet

When the bad news came through from that blunt Australian doctor in Woolloomoolloo — "Keep this up and you've got two years at the most" — Myra decided I had to go on a rigid but sensible diet. She got in touch with Patricia Dunne-North, a dietician who runs her own slimming clubs and to whom Myra had gone in the past for herself.

Patricia gave us the diet she has used most successfully in her clubs. It is a sixteen-week diet and every meal is planned out for you, so that each day's food provides a perfect chemical balance. You don't even have the worry of wondering, "What on earth can I allow myself to eat today?" It is all there for you.

Because the diet is chemically worked out, you *must* eat all the food you are allotted for each day. No cutting back or skipping meals. It isn't even necessary. Patricia tells me that people have lost up to five and a half stone in four months by keeping religiously to her diet. And you can see for yourself that the diet allows you plenty to eat.

"You never go hungry on this diet," says Patricia. "That's the best thing about it."

You are allowed to substitute different vegetables and different types of fish for those on the menu — if you choose from the list that is provided before the diet menus section. Where no quantity is given on the menus for vegetables, you can eat as much as you like, as long as you don't exceed 14 oz a day — and that is a lot. If you are going to stick to the diet to the letter, be sure to follow the special rules that are listed on pages 39 and 40.

I have to admit that Myra and I made some adaptations to the diet, which is why I didn't lose quite as much weight as quickly as I might have. But knowing myself, I realised it would work better for me if I allowed myself a few changes that would make it easier for me to stick to the diet in the long run. So Myra and I drank skimmed milk in coffee but not in tea — but made sure we had fewer cups than we used to.

I can't bear low-fat spreads so Myra would put butter on my toast and then scrape it off again. And cottage cheese was out for me. I loathe it.

The other personal decision I made was to cut out potatoes completely. I'm a potatoholic, if there is such a thing. I only have to have one and I want sixteen more. The very taste sets me off on an enormous craving. I decided that I could only mangage if I said no to beloved potatoes forever and Patricia agreed that would be all right if I substituted rice or bread. I had, of course, to deviate from the diet when I was away, which was very often. But even then it was easier than I thought to keep to the spirit of the thing.

The best thing about the diet, of course, was not going hungry, even though some of my favourite things were out. But some of my favourites were left in too — I'm partial to a roast and there are all kinds of roasts allowed on Sundays. Even roast lamb. We don't have roast shoulder any more, because Myra insists it's too fattening, but we both enjoy roast leg of lamb instead, cooked slowly to make it tender and full of flavour.

Of course I of all people am not claiming it is easy to change the bad food habits of a lifetime overnight. But it is so much easier if you have the real will to win.

Diet rules

Don't swap

Each day's meals are carefully planned to give a proper balance of the various food elements. You can substitute one type of fish for another (see page 41), but not — say — fish for meat. Don't swap meals around by eating Wednesday's breakfast and Saturday's lunch. Tick off days as you complete them.

Quantities

The quantities given are for women. Teenagers (those up to 16) should take 4 oz dried milk, or 1 pint skimmed milk daily; and an extra 2 slices of bread. Teenagers and men must add two more fruits a day to the basic diet. Men should also add 2 oz extra fish and meat, and an extra 2 slices of bread.

Weights

All the weights given in the diet are of food ready to eat. By and large, you can calculate that things will lose 2 oz in cooking; if a piece of meat contains bone, a rough guide is to allow 2 oz for that also. Thus, to end up with a 6 oz cooked chop, you should ask the butcher for one weighing 10 oz. The easiest way to weigh out quantities accurately is to use scales (the sort with a dial are probably easier to use than those with weights) on which you can balance your plate. Once you know how much the plate weighs, you can add vegetables and meat or fish to the correct amounts. Warm the plate first for a hot meal.

Milk

Either use a pint of skimmed milk a day, or take 2 oz daily of a powdered milk such as Marvel. When people gain weight, the skin stretches; when they lose it there is a danger of its losing its elasticity. The milk helps to avoid this. One way of taking 2 oz of powdered milk is to have it all at once as a hot bedtime drink, making it up to no less than half a pint.

Other drinks

You are allowed as much tea or coffee as you like, and not only at breakfast time. Drink it black, or (tea) with lemon, or use milk from your daily allowance. Sweeten with a sugar substitute if you must; though it is better to retain a sweet tooth. You are also allowed any 'slimline' drink (low-calorie tonic or bitter lemon, for instance), or low-calorie diet drink, such as Diet Pepsi or Tab. Or soda water, or PLJ ... Something such as this, or tea or coffee, is what 'drink' signifies in lunch and dinner menus. *It does not mean an alcoholic drink.*

Bread
Use ordinary brown or white bread, not a slimming bread and not wholemeal or granary-type bread. Women have 2 oz daily where stated; men and teenagers more (see *Quantities*, above).

Margarine
Use a sunflower margarine, Flora or any own-brand variety.

Mayonnaise
Use Mayonnaise, *not* salad cream; not even a special 'slimmers' type. Any good bottled variety of mayonnaise you like will do.

Fruit
Sweeten stewed rhubarb with a sugar substitute. If you choose berries, 5 oz is equivalent to one fruit. No bananas are allowed until Week 7. Avocado pears are not allowed at all.

Vegetables: any amount

Asparagus
Beansprouts
Broccoli
Cabbage, raw, braised, steamed, pickled, stuffed, boiled or tinned
Cauliflower, raw or cooked
Celery, raw or braised, fresh or tinned
Chicory
Courgettes
Cucumber
Endive
Gherkins

Lettuce, all kinds
Marrow
Mushrooms, raw or cooked, fresh or tinned
Mustard and cress
Peppers, red or green
Radishes
Runner beans
Spring greens
Spinach
Tomatoes, fresh or tinned, and juice
Turnip tops
Watercress

Vegetables: only 4 oz daily

Artichokes
Bamboo shoots
Beetroot
Broad beans
Brussels sprouts
Carrots, raw or cooked
Leeks

Onions
Peas
Parsnips
Spring onions
Swede
Sweet corn
Turnips

Cereals: only 1 oz daily

All-Bran
Bran Flakes
Cornflakes
Instant oatmeal
Puffed Wheat
Quick Quaker Oats
Rice Krispies

Rolled oats
Shredded Wheat
Shreddies
Special K
Weetabix
Wheat flakes

Permitted fish (for substitution)

Bass: grill, poach or bake; 'dry fry' small whole fish
Brill: 'dry fry' fillets poach or bake whole fish and fillets
Cod: grill, poach or bake
Coley: grill, poach or bake
Haddock: dry fry, poach; if smoked, poach
Hake: grill or poach
Halibut: poach
Mackerel: grill or poach; if tinned, drain off the oil
Plaice: 'dry fry', grill or poach
Salmon: poach, grill or bake; if smoked, eat raw: if tinned, drain off the oil
Tuna: grill, poach or bake; if tinned, drain off the oil

	Breakfast	Lunch	Dinner
MONDAY	5 oz grapefruit segments 1 boiled egg 1 slice toast tea or coffee	4 oz tinned tuna fish lettuce sliced tomatoes sliced cucumber 1 slice bread 1 tsp margarine 1 apple drink	6 oz chicken 4 oz peas cauliflower 8 oz stewed rhubarb drink
TUESDAY	4 fl oz fruit juice 1 oz hard cheese 1 slice bread tea or coffee	4 oz grilled haddock green beans 1 slice bread 1 tsp margarine 1 apple drink	6 oz tinned salmon mixed salad 2 oz beetroot 2 oz spring onions 2 tsps mayonnaise 1 fruit drink
WEDNESDAY	2 oz prunes 1 oz cereal tea or coffee	4 oz tinned mackerel sliced tomatoes sliced cucumber chicory 1 slice bread 3 tsps margarine 1 fruit drink	6 oz grilled pork chop 3 oz potatoes 4 oz peas cauliflower 1 fruit drink
THURSDAY	4 fl oz fruit juice 2 oz cottage cheese 1 slice bread tea or coffee	4 oz sardines 1 slice toast mixed salad 2 oz beetroot 1 tblsp mayonnaise 1 fruit (apple) drink	6 oz chicken 2 oz sprouts green beans 1 orange drink

week 1

	Breakfast	**Lunch**	**Dinner**
FRIDAY	1 apple 1 oz cereal tea or coffee	1 roll 6 oz corned beef 2 tsps mayonnaise 1 tsp margarine lettuce cucumber chicory 1 fruit drink	2-egg omelette mushrooms tomatoes cauliflower 3 oz potatoes 1 orange drink
SATURDAY	1 orange 1 scrambled egg 1 slice toast tea or coffee	4 oz grilled liver 2 oz peas 2 oz carrots 1 slice bread 3 tsps margarine 1 fruit drink	6 oz fish green beans cauliflower 1 fruit drink
SUNDAY	4 fl oz fruit juice 1 oz cereal tea or coffee	6 oz roast lamb 3 oz jacket potato 2 oz sprouts 2 oz peas 1 orange drink	4 oz tinned pilchards green salad (no onions) 1 slice bread 2 tsps mayonnaise 1 tsp margarine 1 fruit drink

Note: Use 1 pint skimmed milk daily or 2 oz powdered milk

Teenagers (those up to 16): Add 2 oz skimmed milk per day
: Add 2 extra slices bread per day
: Add 2 extra fruits per day

Men: Add 2 extra slices bread per day
: Add 2 oz extra fish and meat per day
: Add 2 extra fruits per day

	Breakfast	**Lunch**	**Dinner**
MONDAY	4 fl oz fruit juice 1 poached egg 1 slice toast 2 tsps margarine tea or coffee	4 oz chicken lettuce tomatoes celery 1 slice bread 1 tsp margarine 1 fruit drink	6 oz grilled lamb chop 2 oz peas 2 oz swede 1 fruit drink
TUESDAY	1 orange 1 oz cereal tea or coffee	2-egg omelette mushrooms tomatoes 1 slice bread 3 tsps margarine 1 apple drink	6 oz grilled veal broccoli 4 oz peas 3 oz potatoes 1 fruit drink
WEDNESDAY	½ grapefruit 1 oz hard cheese 1 slice toast tea or coffee	4 oz poached whiting cauliflower 1 slice bread 3 tsps margarine 1 fruit drink	6 oz liver casseroled in tomato juice with 2 oz onions 2 oz carrots tomatoes fruit drink
THURSDAY	4 fl oz fruit juice 1 oz cereal tea or cereal	4 oz tinned tuna fish sliced cucumber sliced tomatoes celery 1 tblsp mayonnaise 1 fruit drink	6 oz roast chicken 3 oz jacket potato 2 oz carrots 2 oz peas 1 fruit drink

week 2

	Breakfast	Lunch	Dinner
FRIDAY	1 apple 1 scrambled egg 1 slice toast 1 tsp margarine tea or coffee	4 oz tinned pilchards 1 slice bread 2 tsps mayonnaise lettuce tomatoes chicory 1 fruit drink	6 oz grilled beefburger 4 oz sprouts spring cabbage 1 fruit drink
SATURDAY	4 fl oz orange juice 2 oz cottage cheese 1 slice toast tea or coffee	4 oz grilled haddock green beans cauliflower 1 slice bread 3 tsps margarine fruit drink	6 oz pork chop 4 oz sprouts grilled tomatoes 1 fruit drink
SUNDAY	½ grapefruit 1 oz cereal tea or coffee	6 oz roast chicken 3 oz jacket potato 2 oz swede 2 oz peas 8 oz stewed rhubarb drink	2 oz hard cheese lettuce sliced tomatoes chicory celery 1 apple drink

Note: Use 1 pint skimmed milk daily or 2 oz powdered milk
Teenagers (those up to 16): Add 2 oz skimmed milk per day
                        : Add 2 extra slices bread per day
                        : Add 2 extra fruits per day
Men: Add 2 extra slices bread per day
    : Add 2 oz extra fish and meat per day
    : Add 2 extra fruits per day

Menu

	Breakfast	Lunch	Dinner
MONDAY	4 fl oz fruit juice 1 boiled egg 1 slice bread 1 tsp margarine tea or coffee	6 oz ham 4 oz sprouts spring greens 1 fruit drink	4 oz tuna fish celery, tomato and cucumber salad 1 slice bread ½ tsp margarine drink
TUESDAY	1 orange 2 oz cottage cheese 1 slice bread tea or coffee	4 oz mackerel salad 1 slice bread 1 tsp mayonnaise 2 tsps margarine 1 apple drink	6 oz grilled liver 4 oz peas cauliflower 1 fruit drink
WEDNESDAY	1 apple 1 oz cereal tea or coffee	2-egg omelette 4 oz peas 1 slice bread 3 tsps margarine 1 fruit drink	6 oz grilled pork spinach 1 fruit drink
THURSDAY	fruit 1 poached egg 1 slice bread 1 tsp margarine tea or coffee	mixed salad 2 oz hard cheese 2 tsps mayonnaise 1 fruit drink	6 oz grilled veal 3 oz baked potato 4 oz sprouts 1 fruit drink

week 3

	Breakfast	Lunch	Dinner
FRIDAY	*4 oz tomato juice* *1 oz hard cheese* *1 slice bread* *tea or coffee*	*4 oz sardines* *4 oz raw carrots* *green salad* *1 tblsp mayonnaise* *1 fruit* *drink*	*6 oz grilled cod with* *lemon juice* *3 oz rice* *green beans* *1 fruit* *drink*
SATURDAY	*4 fl oz fruit juice* *1 oz cereal* *tea or coffee*	*6 oz roast lamb* *spring greens* *3 oz potato* *1 fruit* *drink*	*4 oz tinned salmon* *mixed salad* *1 tblsp oil or vinegar* *1 fruit* *drink*
SUNDAY	*1 pear* *2 oz hard cheese* *1 slice bread* *½ tsp margarine* *tea or coffee*	*6 oz roast chicken* *cabbage* *4 oz peas* *fruit juice*	*4 oz cold beef* *1 slice bread* *½ tsp margarine* *mixed salad* *2 tsps mayonnaise* *tomatoes* *1 fruit* *drink*

Note: Use 1 pint skimmed milk daily or 2 oz powdered milk
Teenagers (those up to 16): Add 2 oz skimmed milk per day
                             : Add 2 extra slices bread per day
                             : Add 2 extra fruits per day
Men: Add 2 extra slices bread per day
   : Add 2 oz extra fish and meat per day
   : Add 2 extra fruits per day

	Breakfast	Lunch	Dinner
MONDAY	4 fl oz orange drink 1 oz hard cheese 1 slice bread tea or coffee	4 oz chicken liver pâté 1 slice toast mixed salad 1 tblsp mayonnaise 1 fruit drink	6 oz chicken broccoli 4 oz sprouts 1 fruit drink
TUESDAY	1 orange 1 oz cereal tea or coffee	cauliflower with 2 oz cheese 1 slice bread 3 tsps margarine 1 fruit drink	6 oz grilled liver 3 oz potatoes 4 oz onions 1 fruit drink
WEDNESDAY	½ medium grapefruit 1 poached egg 1 slice bread 2 tsps margarine tea or coffee	4 oz smoked haddock green beans 1 slice bread 1 tsp margarine fruit drink	6 oz grilled lamb chop 4 oz swede cabbage fruit drink
THURSDAY	8 fl oz tomato juice 2 oz cottage cheese 1 slice bread 1 tsp margarine tea or coffee	mushroom and 2-egg omelette 1 slice bread 2 tsps margarine fruit drink	6 oz grilled veal 4 oz sprouts fruit drink

week 4

	Breakfast	**Lunch**	**Dinner**
FRIDAY	5 oz tinned grapefruit 1 oz cereal tea or coffee	4 oz tinned tuna fish green salad 1 slice bread 3 tsps margarine fruit drink	6 oz grilled chicken 3 oz potatoes 2 oz peas 2 oz carrots fruit drink
SATURDAY	1 apple 1 scrambled egg 2 slices bread 3 tsps margarine tea or coffee	4 oz grilled cod 4 oz peas 1 orange drink	6 oz grilled beefburgers grilled mushrooms grilled tomatoes fruit drink
SUNDAY	2 oz prunes 1 oz cereal tea or coffee	6 oz roast beef 3 oz jacket potato cauliflower 4 oz peas fruit drink	4 oz ham mixed salad (no onions, no beetroot) 1 tblsp mayonnaise 1 slice bread fruit drink

Note: Use 1 pint skimmed milk daily or 2 oz powdered milk
Teenagers (those up to 16): Add 2 oz skimmed milk per day
: Add 2 extra slices bread per day
: Add 2 extra fruits per day
Men: Add 2 extra slices bread per day
: Add 2 oz extra fish and meat per day
: Add 2 extra fruits per day

Menu

	Breakfast	**Lunch**	**Dinner**
MONDAY	4 fl oz orange juice 1 oz hard cheese 1 slice bread 1 tsp margarine tea or coffee	4 oz smoked haddock cauliflower 1 slice bread 2 tsps margarine fruit drink	6 oz grilled liver 4 oz carrots cabbage 1 fruit drink
TUESDAY	5 cubes melon 1 oz cereal tea or coffee	4 oz ham 3 oz potatoes mixed green salad (no onions, no beetroot) 2 tsps mayonnaise 1 apple drink	6 oz grilled cod green beans 4 oz peas 1 slice bread 1 tsp margarine fruit drink
WEDNESDAY	4 fl oz fruit juice 1 boiled egg 1 slice bread 1 tsp margarine tea or coffee	4 oz mackerel 4 oz butter beans 1 slice bread 2 tsps margarine fruit drink	6 oz chicken green beans cabbage fruit drink
THURSDAY	½ grapefruit 1 oz cereal tea or coffee	4 oz cottage cheese tomatoes 1 slice bread 3 tsps margarine fruit drink	6 oz grilled pork chop 4 oz sprouts 3 oz potatoes fruit drink

week 5

	Breakfast	Lunch	Dinner
FRIDAY	1 orange 1 poached egg 1 slice bread 1 tsp margarine tea or coffee	4 fl oz tomato juice 2 oz hard cheese 1 tblsp mayonnaise green salad 1 slice bread fruit drink	6 oz grilled white fish 4 oz butter beans fruit drink
SATURDAY	½ grapefruit 1 scrambled egg with tomato 1 slice toast tea or coffee	4 oz sardines mixed green salad 1 tblsp mayonnaise 1 slice bread fruit drink	6 oz grilled beefburger 4 oz carrots cabbage fruit drink
SUNDAY	orange juice 1 oz cereal tea or coffee	6 oz grilled steak cabbage 4 oz peas 3 oz jacket potato drink	2-egg omelette with mushrooms and tomatoes 1 fruit 1 slice bread 3 tsps margarine drink

Note: Use 1 pint skimmed milk daily or 2 oz powdered milk

Teenagers (those up to 16): Add 2 oz skimmed milk per day
: Add 2 extra slices bread per day
: Add 2 extra fruits per day

Men: Add 2 extra slices bread per day
: Add 2 oz extra fish and meat per day
: Add 2 extra fruits per day

Menu

	Breakfast	**Lunch**	**Dinner**
MONDAY	*4 fl oz orange juice* *1 oz cereal* *tea or coffee*	*4 oz tinned salmon* *mixed salad* *2 tsps mayonnaise* *1 slice bread* *1 tsp margarine* *fruit* *drink*	*6 oz grilled beefburger* *4 oz peas* *3 oz jacket potato* *fruit* *drink*
TUESDAY	*1 orange* *1 boiled egg* *1 slice toast* *1 tsp margarine* *tea or coffee*	*4 oz poached whiting* *grilled tomatoes* *1 slice bread* *3 tsps margarine* *1 apple* *drink*	*6 oz corned beef* *2 oz carrots* *2 oz peas* *fruit* *drink*
WEDNESDAY	*½ grapefruit* *1 scrambled egg* *1 slice bread* *tea or coffee*	*4 oz ham* *mixed salad* *4 oz onions* *2 tsps mayonnaise* *1 slice bread* *1 tsp margarine* *fruit* *drink*	*6 oz grilled cod* *green beans* *broccoli* *fruit* *drink*
THURSDAY	*8 fl oz tomato juice* *1 oz cereal* *tea or coffee*	*4 oz poached haddock* *poached mushrooms* *1 slice bread* *3 tsps margarine* *1 orange* *drink*	*6 oz grilled pork* *3 oz jacket potato* *4 oz broad beans* *fruit* *drink*

week 6

	Breakfast	Lunch	Dinner
FRIDAY	½ grapefruit 1 oz hard cheese 1 slice bread tea or coffee	4 oz tinned tuna green salad 2 tsps mayonnaise 1 slice bread 1 tsp margarine fruit drink	6 oz chicken 4 oz peas green beans fruit drink
SATURDAY	4 fl oz orange juice 2 oz cottage cheese 1 slice bread tea or coffee	6 oz roast chicken 4 oz sprouts 1 fruit drink	2-egg omelette green salad (no onions, no beetroot) 1 tblsp mayonnaise 1 slice bread drink
SUNDAY	8 fl oz tomato juice 1 oz cereal tea or coffee	6 oz roast lamb 3 oz jacket potato green beans cabbage fruit drink	4 oz tinned pilchards 2 tsps mayonnaise 4 oz peas cauliflower 1 slice bread 1 tsp margarine fruit drink

Note: Use 1 pint skimmed milk daily or 2 oz powdered milk
Teenagers (those up to 16): Add 2 oz skimmed milk per day
                       : Add 2 extra slices bread per day
                       : Add 2 extra fruits per day
Men: Add 2 extra slices bread per day
   : Add 2 oz extra fish and meat per day
   : Add 2 extra fruits per day

Menu

	Breakfast	Lunch	Dinner
MONDAY	1 apple 1 oz hard cheese 1 slice bread 1 tsp margarine tea or coffee	4 oz cold beef 4 oz swede 1 slice bread 2 tsps margarine 1 orange drink	6 oz grilled cod green beans 8 oz stewed rhubarb drink
TUESDAY	1 orange 1 boiled egg 1 slice toast 1 tsp margarine tea or coffee	4 oz cottage cheese tomatoes cold or grilled 1 slice bread 2 tsps margarine fruit drink	6 oz grilled lamb chop 4 oz peas green beans fruit drink
WEDNESDAY	4 fl oz orange juice 1 oz cereal tea or coffee	mushroom and 2-egg omelette green beans 1 slice bread 3 tsps margarine fruit drink	6 oz grilled steak 3 oz jacket potato 2 oz peas 2 oz carrotss fruit drink

THURSDAY	½ grapefruit
	2 oz cottage cheese
	1 slice toast
	tea or coffee
		4 oz tinned mackerel
		1 tblsp mayonnaise
		tomato salad
		1 slice bread
		fruit
		drink
			6 oz liver, casseroled
			  with 2 oz onions
			  and 2 oz carrots
			cabbage
			1 banana
			drink

week 7

	Breakfast	Lunch	Dinner
FRIDAY	1 apple 1 scrambled egg 1 slice bread tea or coffee	4 oz poached haddock poached mushrooms 3 tsps margarine 1 slice bread 1 fruit (apple) drink	6 oz roast chicken broccoli 4 oz peas fruit drink
SATURDAY	4 fl oz fruit juice 1 oz cereal tea or coffee	4 oz ham 1 slice bread 3 tsps margarine green salad 4 oz onions fruit drink	4 oz poached whiting grilled tomatoes cauliflower 3 oz potatoes 1 apple drink
SUNDAY	8 fl oz tomato juice 1 oz cereal tea or coffee	4 oz roast beef 4 oz roast onions 3 oz jacket potato green beans fruit drink	4 oz tuna fish 2 tsps mayonnaise mixed green salad 1 slice bread 1 tsp margarine fruit drink

Note: Use 1 pint skimmed milk daily or 2 oz powdered milk
Teenagers (those up to 16): Add 2 oz skimmed milk per day
                                : Add 2 extra slices bread per day
                                : Add 2 extra fruits per day
Men: Add 2 extra slices bread per day
    : Add 2 oz extra fish and meat per day
    : Add 2 extra fruits per day

Menu

	Breakfast	**Lunch**	**Dinner**
MONDAY	½ grapefruit 1 egg 1 slice bread 1 tsp margarine tea or coffee	4 oz tinned tuna fish tomato and lettuce salad 1 slice bread ½ tsp margarine 1 apple drink	6 oz roast chicken 4 oz peas cabbage 1 orange drink
TUESDAY	4 fl oz orange juice 1 oz cereal tea or coffee	4 oz cottage cheese cucumber and tomato 2 oz beetroot ½ oz margarine 1 slice bread 1 orange drink	6 oz grilled steak 2 oz onions 3 oz jacket potato 8 oz stewed rhubarb drink
WEDNESDAY	8 fl oz tomato juice 1 scrambled egg 1 slice toast tea or coffee	4 oz poached haddock mushrooms 1 slice bread 3 tsps margarine 1 fruit drink	6 oz grilled veal 4 oz carrots 1 fruit drink
THURSDAY	4 fl oz fruit juice 1 oz cereal tea or coffee	2 oz cheese green salad (no onions, no beetroot) 1 tblsp mayonnaise fruit drink	6 oz grilled pork chop 4 oz sprouts 3 oz potatoes fruit drink

week 8

	Breakfast	**Lunch**	**Dinner**

FRIDAY	8 fl oz tomato juice
	1 oz hard cheese
	1 slice toast
	tea or coffee
		2-egg omelette with
		   mushrooms and
		   tomatoes
		1 slice bread
		3 tsps margarine
		fruit
		drink
			6 oz ham
			mixed salad with
			   2 oz spring onions
			   2 oz beetroot
			fruit
			drink

SATURDAY	4 fl oz fruit juice 1 oz cereal tea or coffee	4 oz poached cod green beans 1 slice bread 3 tsps margarine fruit drink	6 oz grilled liver 4 oz peas 3 oz potatoes fruit drink
SUNDAY	½ grapefruit 1 oz hard cheese 1 slice toast tea or coffee	6 oz roast lamb 2 oz peas 2 oz roast parsnips fruit drink	4 oz tinned salmon green salad 1 slice bread 3 tsps margarine fruit drink

Note: Use 1 pint skimmed milk daily or 2 oz powdered milk
Teenagers (those up to 16): Add 2 oz skimmed milk per day
                    : Add 2 extra slices bread per day
                    : Add 2 extra fruits per day
Men: Add 2 extra slices bread per day
   : Add 2 oz extra fish and meat per day
   : Add 2 extra fruits per day

Menu

	Breakfast	Lunch	Dinner
MONDAY	½ grapefruit 1 egg 1 slice bread 2 tsps margarine tea or coffee	4 oz tuna fish lettuce and tomato salad 1 slice bread 1 tsp margarine fruit drink	6 oz grilled chicken 4 oz peas 2 only tinned plums drink
TUESDAY	8 fl oz tomato juice 1 oz cereal tea or coffee	4 oz chicken mixed salad (no onions, no beetroot) 1 tbslp mayonnaise fruit drink	6 oz grilled beefburger 4 oz peas 3 oz potatoes fruit drink
WEDNESDAY	1 slice unsweetened pineapple 2 oz cottage cheese 1 slice bread tea or coffee	4 oz mackerel, tomato and cucumber salad 1 slice bread 3 tsps margarine fruit drink	6 oz ham cauliflower broad beans fruit drink
THURSDAY	1 apple 1 oz cereal tea or coffee	4 oz sardines on toast 3 tsps margarine shredded cabbage pickled cucumber 1 fruit drink	6 oz grilled lamb chop 3 oz jacket potato 4 oz carrots fruit drink

week 9

	Breakfast	Lunch	Dinner

FRIDAY	1 orange
	scrambled egg on toast
	tea or coffee
		2 oz hard cheese
		green mixed salad
		1 slice bread
		1 tsp margarine
		2 tsps mayonnaise
		fruit
		drink
			6 oz grilled liver and
			  4 oz onions or
			  liver and onion
			  casseroled in tomato
			  juice
			fruit
			drink

SATURDAY	4 fl oz fruit juice
	1 oz hard cheese
	  on 1 slice toast
		6 oz grilled pork chop
		green beans
		4 oz peas
		fruit
		drink
			mushroom and 2-egg
			  omelette
			3 tsps margarine
			spinach
			fruit
			drink

SUNDAY	8 fl oz tomato juice 1 oz cereal tea or coffee	6 oz roast chicken marrow cabbage 3 oz jacket potato fruit drink	4 oz tinned tuna 1 tblsp mayonnaise mixed salad 2 oz spring onions 2 oz beetroot fruit drink

Note: Use 1 pint skimmed milk daily or 2 oz powdered milk
Teenagers (those up to 16): Add 2 oz skimmed milk per day
                               : Add 2 extra slices bread per day
                               : Add 2 extra fruits per day
Men: Add 2 extra slices bread per day
     : Add 2 oz extra fish and meat per day
     : Add 2 extra fruits per day

Menu

	Breakfast	**Lunch**	**Dinner**
MONDAY	5 oz grapefruit segments 1 oz cereal tea or coffee	2 oz hard cheese 1 roll 1 tblsp mayonnaise green salad fruit drink	6 oz chicken broccoli 3 oz potatoes fruit drink
TUESDAY	1 orange 2 oz cottage cheese 1 slice toast tea or coffee	4 oz sardines sliced tomatoes and cucumber 2 tsps mayonnaise 1 slice bread 1 tsp margarine 1 fruit drink	6 oz grilled beefburger 4 oz carrots fruit drink
WEDNESDAY	8 fl oz tomato juice 1 boiled egg 1 slice bread 1 tsp margarine tea or coffee	4 oz grilled haddock poached mushrooms 1 slice bread 1 tsp margarine 1 orange drink	6 oz casseroled liver and 4 oz onions cabbage green beans apple drink
THURSDAY	1 apple 1 scrambled egg 1 slice toast tea or coffee	4 oz tinned tuna fish 1 slice bread 1 tsp margarine lettuce cucumber celery 2 tsps mayonnaise 1 orange drink	6 oz lamb chop 4 oz peas cauliflower fruit drink

week 10

	Breakfast	**Lunch**	**Dinner**
FRIDAY	2 oz prunes 1 oz cereal tea or coffee	4 oz tinned salmon 1 slice bread 3 tsps margarine tomatoes 4 oz spring onions fruit drink	6 oz chicken 3 oz jacket potato broccoli cauliflower fruit
SATURDAY	fruit juice 1 oz hard cheese 1 slice bread 1 tsp margarine tea or coffee	2-egg omelette grilled tomatoes 1 slice bread 2 tsps margarine fruit drink	6 oz grilled veal 4 oz swede cabbage fruit drink
SUNDAY	5 oz grapefruit segments 1 oz cereal tea or coffee	6 oz roast pork 3 oz jacket potato 2 oz boiled parsnips 2 oz peas 8 oz stewed rhubarb drink	4 oz tinned salmon lettuce and tomato salad 1 tblsp mayonnaise 1 apple drink

Note: Use 1 pint skimmed milk daily or 2 oz powdered milk
Teenagers (those up to 16): Add 2 oz skimmed milk per day
: Add 2 extra slices bread per day
: Add 2 extra fruits per day
Men: Add 2 extra slices bread per day
: Add 2 oz extra fish and meat per day
: Add 2 extra fruits per day

Menu

	Breakfast	Lunch	Dinner
MONDAY	4 fl oz fruit juice 1 scrambled egg 1 slice bread ½ tsp margarine tea or coffee	4 oz smoked haddock poached mushrooms 1 slice bread 1 tsp margarine 1 apple drink	6 oz chicken 4 oz peas broccoli 1 orange drink
TUESDAY	1 orange 1 oz cereal tea or coffee	4 oz cold chicken green salad (no onions, no beetroot) 1 tblsp mayonnaise fruit drink	6 oz grilled trout tomatoes 3 oz potatoes 4 oz leeks fruit drink
WEDNESDAY	½ grapefruit 2 oz cottage cheese 1 slice toast tea or coffee	4 oz tinned tuna fish sliced cucumber celery 1 slice bread 3 tsps margarine fruit drink	6 oz grilled liver green beans 4 oz peas fruit drink
THURSDAY	8 fl oz tomato juice 1 boiled egg 1 slice bread ½ tsp margarine tea or coffee	2-egg omelette mushrooms and tomatoes 1 slice bread 1 tsp margarine fruit drink	6 oz grilled steak 4 oz carrots greens fruit drink

week 11

	Breakfast	Lunch	Dinner
FRIDAY	1 apple 1 oz cereal tea or coffee	2 oz hard cheese lettuce 2 oz spring onions 2 oz beetroot 3 oz cold potato 1 tblsp mayonnaise fruit drink	6 oz grilled pork chop green beans cabbage fruit drink
SATURDAY	4 fl oz fruit juice 1 oz hard cheese 1 slice toast tea or coffee	6 oz ham 4 oz peas 1 slice bread 3 tsps margarine fruit drink	4 oz poached whiting green beans cauliflower fruit drink
SUNDAY	8 fl oz tomato juice 1 oz cereal tea or coffee	6 oz roast lamb broccoli cauliflower 3 oz potatoes mint sauce fruit drink	4 oz sardines mixed salad 2 oz beetroot 2 oz carrots 1 tblsp mayonnaise fruit drink

Note: Use 1 pint skimmed milk daily or 2 oz powdered milk

Teenagers (those up to 16): Add 2 oz skimmed milk per day
                           : Add 2 extra slices bread per day
                           : Add 2 extra fruits per day

Men: Add 2 extra slices bread per day
    : Add 2 oz extra fish and meat per day
    : Add 2 extra fruits per day

Menu

	Breakfast	**Lunch**	**Dinner**
MONDAY	4 fl oz orange juice 1 boiled egg 1 slice toast 1 tsp margarine tea or coffee	4 oz tuna fish 2 tsps mayonnaise 4 oz beetroot 1 slice bread 1 apple drink	4 oz mixed vegetable juice 6 oz ham spring greens 1 orange drink
TUESDAY	1 apple 2 oz cottage cheese 1 slice bread tea or coffee	4 oz canned mackerel mixed salad 2 tsps mayonnaise 1 slice bread fruit drink	6 oz grilled liver 4 oz green onions cauliflower fruit drink
WEDNESDAY	½ grapefruit 1 oz cereal tea or coffee	2 hard boiled eggs with green salad 1 slice bread ½ oz margarine fruit drink	6 oz grilled pork chop 3 oz rice spinach 4 oz peas fruit drink
THURSDAY	8 fl oz tomato juice 1 oz hard cheese 1 slice bread tea or coffee	4 oz sardines sliced tomatoes sliced cucumber 1 slice bread ½ oz margarine fruit drink	grilled veal 2 oz carrots 2 oz peas fruit drink

week 12

	Breakfast	Lunch	Dinner
FRIDAY	1 orange 1 oz cereal tea or coffee	4 oz pilchards green salad tomatoes fruit 1 slice bread ½ oz margarine drink	6 oz smoked haddock 3 oz boiled potatoes 4 oz peas green beans fruit drink
SATURDAY	1 apple 1 scrambled egg 1 slice toast tea or coffee	6 oz chicken 4 oz sprouts marrow or cauliflower 1 orange drink	4 oz poached cod 1 slice bread ½ ox margarine green beans fruit drink
SUNDAY	3 dried prunes 1 oz cereal tea or coffee	6 oz roast beef 3 oz potatoes cabbage marrow or green beans fruit drink	2 oz hard cheese tossed salad 2 oz spring onions 2 oz beetroot 1 slice bread 3 tsps margarine fruit drink

Note: Use 1 pint skimmed milk daily or 2 oz powdered milk
Teenagers (those up to 16): Add 2 oz skimmed milk per day
: Add 2 extra slices bread per day
: Add 2 extra fruits per day
Men: Add 2 extra slices bread per day
: Add 2 oz extra fish and meat per day
: Add 2 extra fruits per day

Menu

	Breakfast	**Lunch**	**Dinner**
MONDAY	4 fl oz fruit juice 1 boiled egg 1 slice bread 1 tsp margarine tea or coffee	4 oz tinned salmon mixed salad 1 slice bread 2 tsps margarine 1 orange drink	6 oz corned beef 4 oz broad beans fruit drink
TUESDAY	1 orange 1 oz cereal tea or coffee	4 oz cottage cheese celery tomato and cucumber 1 tblsp mayonnaise 1 slice bread fruit drink	6 oz grilled pork 4 oz peas 3 oz jacket potato fruit drink
WEDNESDAY	8 fl oz tomato juice 2 oz cottage cheese 1 tomato tea or coffee	4 oz tinned mackerel 2 tsps mayonnaise 2 oz beetroot 2 oz onions 1 slice bread 1 tsp margarine fruit drink	6 oz ham green beans cauliflower fruit drink
THURSDAY	½ grapefruit 1 scrambled egg 1 slice toast tea or coffee	4 oz poached cod poached mushrooms 1 slice bread 3 tsps margarine fruit drink	4 fl oz Campbells V8 vegetable juice 6 oz chicken 4 oz sprouts fruit drink

week 13

	Breakfast	Lunch	Dinner
FRIDAY	4 fl oz fruit juice 1 oz cereal tea or coffee	mushroom and 2-egg omelette 2 slices bread 3 tsps margarine fruit drink	6 oz grilled liver beans 4 oz sprouts fruit drink
SATURDAY	1 apple 1 oz hard cheese 1 slice bread tea or coffee	6 oz roast chicken 4 oz sprouts fruit drink	4 oz baked trout 1 slice bread 3 tsps margarine cauliflower fruit drink
SUNDAY	½ grapefruit 1 oz cereal tea or coffee	6 oz roast lamb 2 oz peas 2 oz sprouts 3 oz potatoes fruit drink	2 oz hard cheese mixed green salad 1 slice bread 3 tsps margarine fruit drink

Note: Use 1 pint skimmed milk daily or 2 oz powdered milk
Teenagers (those up to 16): Add 2 oz skimmed milk per day
: Add 2 extra slices bread per day
: Add 2 extra fruits per day
Men: Add 2 extra slices bread per day
: Add 2 oz extra fish and meat per day
: Add 2 extra fruits per day

$\mathcal{M}$enu

	Breakfast	**Lunch**	**Dinner**
MONDAY	½ grapefruit 2 oz cottage cheese 1 slice toast tea or coffee	4 oz tinned mackerel tomatoes lettuce 2 tsps mayonnaise 1 apple drink	6 oz chicken 4 oz peas green beans fruit drink
TUESDAY	4 fl oz orange juice 1 oz cereal tea or coffee	4 oz cottage cheese celery cucumber 1 slice bread 3 tsps margarine fruit drink	6 oz liver and 4 oz onions casseroled in tomato juice 3 oz potatoes cauliflower fruit drink
WEDNESDAY	1 orange 1 boiled egg 1 slice toast 1 tsp margarine tea or coffee	4 oz poached whiting cauliflower 1 slice bread 2 tsps margarine fruit drink	6 oz grilled veal 4 oz sprouts spring cabbage 8 oz stewed rhubarb fruit drink
THURSDAY	½ grapefruit 1 oz cereal tea or coffee	2 oz hard cheese mixed salad 1 tblsp mayonnaise 1 slice bread fruit drink	6 oz tongue 3 oz potatoes 4 oz peas fruit drink

week 14

	Breakfast	**Lunch**	**Dinner**
FRIDAY	1 apple 1 oz hard cheese 1 slice toast tea or coffee	4 oz chicken sliced cucumber sliced tomato 1 tblsp mayonnaise 1 slice bread 1 orange drink	6 oz poached haddock 4 oz broad beans fruit drink
SATURDAY	4 fl oz fruit juice 1 scrambled egg 1 slice toast tea or coffee	6 oz grilled lamb chop 4 oz sprouts green beans 1 slice bread ½ oz margarine fruit drink	2-egg omelette mushrooms and tomatoes fruit drink
SUNDAY	8 fl oz tomato juice 1 oz cereal tea or coffee	6 oz roast chicken 4 oz swede 3 oz potatoes 1 orange drink	4 oz tinned salmon green salad (no onions, no beetroot) 1 slice bread ½ oz margarine fruit drink

Note: Use 1 pint skimmed milk daily or 2 oz powdered milk
Teenagers (those up to 16): Add 2 oz skimmed milk per day
                     : Add 2 extra slices bread per day
                     : Add 2 extra fruits per day
Men: Add 2 extra slices bread per day
    : Add 2 oz extra fish and meat per day
    : Add 2 extra fruits per day

	Breakfast	**Lunch**	**Dinner**
MONDAY	4 fl oz orange juice	4 oz smoked haddock	6 oz grilled beefburger
	1 poached egg	tomato salad	4 oz onions
	1 slice toast	1 tblsp mayonnaise	fruit
	tea or coffee	fruit	drink
		drink	
TUESDAY	½ grapefruit	2-egg omelette with	6 oz grilled veal
	1 oz cereal	sliced tomatoes	½ oz margarine
	tea or coffee	and mushrooms	4 oz peas
		1 apple	3 oz rice
		drink	spinach
			1 orange
			drink
WEDNESDAY	8 fl oz tomato juice	4 oz tinned mackerel	6 oz grilled liver
	2 oz cottage cheese	green salad	4 oz sprouts
	1 slice toast	1 tblsp mayonnaise	grilled tomatoes
	tea or coffee	fruit	1 apple
		drink	drink
THURSDAY	4 fl oz fruit juice	4 oz tuna fish	6 oz chicken
	1 scrambled egg	1 slice bread	2 oz peas
	1 slice toast	½ oz margarine	spring greens
	tea or coffee	2 oz sliced arrots	8 oz stewed rhubarb
		sliced cucumber	drink
		1 pear	
		drink	

week 15

	Breakfast	Lunch	Dinner
FRIDAY	2 oz prunes 1 oz cereal tea or coffee	2 oz hard cheese 1 roll ½ oz margarine green salad green or red peppers 1 pear drink	4 oz smoked haddock 4 oz peas fruit drink
SATURDAY	4 fl oz fruit juice 1 oz hard cheese 1 slice toast tea of coffee	4 oz tinned salmon pickled cucumber 1 tsp mayonnaise 1 slice bread ½ tsp margarine fruit drink	6 oz chicken green beans cauliflower fruit drink
SUNDAY	1 pear 1 oz cereal tea or coffee	6 oz roast lamb 2 oz leeks 2 oz peas 3 oz jacket potato fruit drink	4 oz sardines 1 slice bread 1 tsp margarine lettuce tomatoes cucumber fruit drink

Note: Use 1 pint skimmed milk daily or 2 oz powdered milk
Teenagers (those up to 16): Add 2 oz skimmed milk per day
                : Add 2 extra slices bread per day
                : Add 2 extra fruits per day
Men: Add 2 extra slices bread per day
   : Add 2 oz extra fish and meat per day
   : Add 2 extra fruits per day

Menu

	Breakfast	Lunch	Dinner
MONDAY	4 fl oz orange juice 1 scrambled egg 1 slice toast tea or coffe	4 oz ham mixed salad 1 tblsp mayonnaise 1 slice bread fruit drink	2-egg omelette mushrooms tomatoes 4 oz peas fruit drink
TUESDAY	½ grapefruit 1 oz cereal tea of coffee	4 oz poached haddock green beans grilled tomatoes 1 slice bread 2 oz margarine fruit drink	6 oz lamb chop 4 oz sprouts 3 oz potatoes fruit drink
WEDNESDAY	4 fl oz fruit juice 2 oz cottage cheese 1 slice toast tea or coffee	4 oz tinned pilchards 1 tblsp mayonnaise tossed salad 4 oz spring onions 1 fruit drink	4 fl oz Campbells V8 vegetable juice 6 oz poached whiting poached mushrooms fruit drink
THURSDAY	8 fl oz tomato juice 1 boiled egg 1 slice bread 1 tsp margarine tea or coffee	4 oz mackerel sliced tomatoes sliced cucumber 1 tsp mayonnaise 1 slice bread fruit drink	6 oz grilled chicken 4 oz sprouts broccoli fruit drink

week 16

	Breakfast	**Lunch**	**Dinner**
FRIDAY	1 apple 1 oz hard cheese 1 slice bread tea or coffee	4 oz tinned salmon green salad green peppers chicory 1 slice bread 1 tblsp mayonnaise fruit drink	grilled cod with lemon juice and parsley 4 oz peas cauliflower fruit drink
SATURDAY	4 fl oz. fruit juice 1 oz cereal tea or coffee	6 oz grilled liver 4 oz sprouts 3 oz potatoes fruit drink	4 oz sardines slice toast mixed salad 1 tsp margarine fruit drink
SUNDAY	1 orange 1 oz cereal tea or coffee	6 oz roast beef 2 oz roast parsnips 2 oz swede 3 oz potatoes fruit drink	2 oz hard cheese 1 slice bread celery lettuce tomatoes 1 tblsp mayonnaise fruit drink

Note: Use 1 pint skimmed milk daily or 2 oz powdered milk
Teenagers (those up to 16): Add 2 oz skimmed milk per day
                : Add 2 extra slices bread per day
                : Add 2 extra fruits per day
Men: Add 2 extra slices bread per day
   : Add 2 oz extra fish and meat per day
   : Add 2 extra fruits per day

Here are a few of my own special tips to help you to be successful, too.

1 No treats

I know it is hard but you just can't afford to indulge yourself at all. Treats are the thin end of the wedge, they lead you back to fatness. We've all done it — "I'll just have this one little chocolate and then no more". But it is slimmer's suicide and we know it. This time round I made a firm commitment with myself that no chocolate, no pastry, no teeny weeny crinkled-up chip would ever pass my lips. Having accepted that, it was so much easier to stick to the straight and narrow. It is possible, I assure you, if you want to succeed strongly enough. Could I, once, ever have believed there was life without potatoes? I now know there is.

2 Don't think of food

That's a hard one during the first couple of weeks. I found my mind straying to the delights of dinners past while drinking my slimline drinks, but that was as far as I ever let it go. It's important to keep youself occupied as much as you can. If you need to do something with your hands, take up knitting or do some carpentry work. And if your mind still goes where you wished it wouldn't go, fill your thoughts with something else instead. Read a book or write a letter — anything that doesn't leave time or space for your fancies to take over. On those rare occasions when I really couldn't banish the ghost of grub, my solution was to study next day's diet menu and find something there to look forward to and focus on instead. But if you do that — make sure you read your diet menu, not a gourmet recipe book or a restaurant menu card.

3 Don't worry about cravings

I wouldn't have believed it possible that I would ever stop

craving for all my favourite forbidden foods. But really, if you stick to your guns, even the strongest cravings disappear after a couple of weeks. I can talk about all my old loves, steak and kidney and spaghetti and chips, with only the faintest whiff of nostalgia now. I've found instead that I actually enjoy foods I wouldn't have dreamt of giving plate room to before. Salads, with tomatoes and lettuce and cucumbers and onions, are something I actually relish now. And apples are almost a treat.

4 Don't bury your head

It helps not to be subjected to tantalising smells and mouth-watering sights when you are starting off on your diet. But it isn't always possible. It is much better to strengthen your resolve to take it like a man (or woman) than to try to organise your life so that you never come eyeball to eyeball with a piece of meringue. If you don't accustom yourself to smelling and seeing without eating, you may not be able to handle the temptation when you do come up against a surprise sausage sizzling in someone else's pan. You can even learn to enjoy smells and sight of foods in a nostalgic martyred sort of way. I'm not saying I haven't sat in restaurants wishing I could be eating the next man's steak and chips instead of my own steamed fish. But I can honestly say now that when I recently went to rehearsals for a television show, which were held in rooms above a restaurant, I did get a righteous vicarious kind of joy from the smell of fried onions wafting up from below.

5 Reward yourself – without food

We all like to give ourselves little presents when we think we've really earned them. I would regularly come off stage after a hard night's singing and gratefully sink into a whisky and soda on the rocks. I felt I'd deserved it. Now I'll put away the soda and ice without the whisky and it is just as refreshing. But if I want a treat, it has got to be something else. A half hour longer in bed, perhaps, or an extravagant item of clothing. The diet is so cheap to eat, you are sure to have extra pennies in your pocket.

6 Don't weigh too often

The temptation to leap on to the bathroom scales every other hour is very difficult to deal with at the beginning. I did it myself and always regretted it later. It means you are looking for instant weight loss and that is not what diets like this are about. Of course, having crept on to the scales, you usually find nothing has happened at all and that can set you into a depression. Worse, you start to wonder if it is even worth carrying on. So bring the scales out just once a week and weigh yourself at the same time of day each time. Don't "have a go" on someone else's scales. They are very likely to be different from your own.

Most important of all, just grit your teeth when you hit the dreaded plateau — that period that seems to last forever when nothing much is shrinking away despite an initial and encouraging shedding of pounds. The lighter you get, the longer it takes to lose weight. So look on the plateau as a register of your success, not a sign of failure.

7 Don't eat too late

If you can avoid it, don't eat your meals too late in the evening. Your digestion is working fastest in the morning, slower in the afternoons and pretty sluggishly by night. But if you are sticking close to Patricia's diet, you needn't worry too much about that. Because it is worked out to provide day-by-day needs exactly, even if you do take your evening meal late, you won't stop losing weight. That is because the meals are not heavy and won't sit in your stomach like lead.

8 Eat three times a day

Make sure you eat breakfast, lunch and dinner, just like it says on the diet sheets. It is the biggest mistake to think that by skipping one meal or putting off eating, you'll do yourself a favour. All you really do is allow your body time to build up a ravenous hunger. You end up starving and it is all the harder then not to dig in and eat much more than you should. Don't starve one day so that you can carry today's meals over to tomorrow and have a real big eat-in. It just doesn't work that way on this diet and you probably won't lose weight if you do it.

9   Don't drink

This diet, in case you haven't noticed, demands abstinence from liquor. It wouldn't be wise to decide to make tiny adaptations to include a glass of wine with lunch or dinner. Alcohol is a bit like chocolate. Once you have one glass of something alcoholic, you get the taste and want to keep having more. That little glass of wine at dinner will soon be urging you towards another little glass at night or a brandy to round off the meal with. Most of us drink not just for the taste but for the feeling it gives us — a loosening up, a relaxation, sometimes even a heady glow and a sense of freedom (of the type that is usually regretted at breakfast next day). If alcohol brings down your social defences, it will probably bring down your food defences too. In the grip of the glow of a spot of wine or whisky, your hand may reach for the roasted peanuts before your heart can stop it.

10   Don't be bullied

You know the scenario. You are at someone else's house for dinner. You have succeeded in politely turning down the avocado with prawns and restricted yourself to a slice of roast and carrots without the creamed potatoes. Then your hostess brings out the chocolate mousse and wheedles, "Oh go on, have some." I can tell you it gets easier to resist when you have a loose waistband to show that your pains to diet have paid off. Nowadays I just pat my slimmed-down belly and say that I am definitely not going to spoil things now. People usually respond to reason and take the plate away. They also respond to authority figures. So tell your host or hostess that your doctor has told you to keep off sweet things completely.

11　Get family support

You can make dieting a kind of a game if you are doing it with someone else. I used to say to Myra, "The first to disappear wins." There is nothing like competition for getting your heart into a diet.

Of course you can't expect everyone else in the house to go on your diet with you, especially if they are wispy slimline types to begin with. But odds are there is at least someone at home who could do with a little compression. And if not, all the more vital to get their moral support for what you are doing. My children were careful not to eat forbidden foods in front of me — and though it wouldn't have thrown me into a salivating froth if they had, it helped me to know that, psychologically, they were with me. Research has shown that women whose husbands take an interest in their reducing diet, and perhaps even keep the score on the scales for them, lose far more weight than those whose husbands are indifferent or downright hostile.

If no one in your family needs to diet but you, try to find someone else with whom to make a slimming pact. I really believe that having a race is a very strong incentive.

12　Make it public

I've said it on television, in the papers and now in this book — I'm never going to be big fat Harry again. I cannot go back on my word now and risk losing face as well as all the health benefits. So tell everyone you know that this diet is the one that's for real and don't pull any punches to give yourself a get-out. Make a commitment in money as well. Start buying the sort of clothes that you will soon be able to fit into. They'll be an incentive to keep on going. The scantier the clothes, the more you seem to have to pay for them nowadays!

Whatever you do, believe in yourself hard enough for others to come to believe in you too. You can hardly abuse their trust and faith by starting to backslide.

Re-educating your appetite

The bonus of the 16-week diet is that it gets you into the right psychological attitude towards food. You will have spent four months eating correctly, perhaps — like me — for the first time in your life. It will be so much easier to adapt that diet to a healthy weight-maintaining way of living.

Not having the right approach is one of the many reasons that starvation and fad diets don't work. I used to try them in the old days: orange diets, pea diets, olive oil and mustard diets. I never usually lasted a day because they were so boring. My stomach wasn't in them, you might say. Even if you do manage to last out the requisite number of days chewing asbestos or whatever your particular fad diet demands, you haven't taught your body to benefit from sensible eating. It will be craving all sorts of things it has been deprived of and you will probably just rush headlong back into all your bad old ways.

Fad diets are a no-no for another reason. They are horrifically unhealthy. You miss out on almost all the essential nutrients that your body requires daily, and as soon as you start to eat again you go back to being two-ton Tessie or Burly Bert.

The only way to lose weight permanently is to lose it slowly and surely and change your eating habits for life. It sounds awfully grim now, perhaps, but once you've got into the swing of it, eating right is as much a habit as eating wrong used to be.

So here are a few tips for changing your eating patterns to make dieting easier on yourself.

1 Make mealtimes your only mealtimes

We all pick up an odd collection of personal eating habits. I know some people who can't eat breakfast sitting down at weekends because they are so used to being in a rush on working mornings.

Try and identify your own special eating habits, those times of day or activities you have come to associate with eating. Do you, for instance, come in from work and relax with a cup of tea and a cake before supper? Do you stop off at the pub for a couple of quick ones? Do you nibble at snacks while doing jobs round the house? Do you like to settle with a book — and a box of chocolates? Do you associate watching TV with dinner on a tray, followed by a non-stop selection of snacks? Do you lunge for the larder whenever you feel miserable or bored?

Whichever questions you answered yes to, it is time to put a stop to that particular habit. The best way to stop eating unconsciously (and if you eat without realising it, that is how you cram the calories in) is to make mealtimes special.

Make a point of sitting down at the table for every meal of the day. If you never have time to sit down to breakfast but just take flying bites of bread and butter as you throw on your clothes and scuttle to the bathroom, you'll have to plan to get up earlier in future.

Don't read the newspaper or work on a problem while you are eating. That just reinforces your habit of connecting reading or working with eating. What you are trying to do is break the connection between eating and any other activity at all. Don't get up from the table until you have finished eating and then, after leaving it, don't eat anything else in any other place in the house. It will take time to get used to, and it might seem a nuisance, but the benefits in saved snatched calories will be enormous. You'll be able to watch television without craving a cream cake and read a novel without one hand in the biscuit tin.

2 Put food away

Don't leave food around where you can see it the moment you walk into the room. Even a filled-up fruit bowl may be more of a temptation than you can stand. You could end up seizing an apple or a pear purely because it has come into your line of vision and not because you are starving for something to eat. Keep bread and spreads wrapped up and out of sight. If you have to have biscuits around the house because your children would scream blue murder without them, put them in a tin and squeeze them right to the back of the furthest food cupboard. If you get the urge to break your diet, by the time you've rooted them out of their hidey-hole, you might have had enough time to regret and not do it.

If you can avoid keeping forbidden foods in the house, do so. You don't need to have biscuits to offer a casual drop-in guest at tea-time. Why not offer them a piece of toast instead?

And don't go shopping when you are feeling hungry. Make a list of what you need that is on your diet sheet and buy only those foods for the day. Don't even look at the other shelves in the supermarket.

3 Don't eat too much of anything

If you are trying to re-educate your appetite, you need to teach yourself to expect *less* food. It is no good satisfying your craving to have something in your mouth by settling for non-stop consumption of low-calorie foods. Too much of anything just allows you to keep right on indulging yourself instead of reducing your old dependence on food. So don't eat piece of fruit after piece of fruit and a stack of vegetables spread out over the day. Learn not to pick and snack. Instead fill yourself up at the right time and not at any other. As I've said, you won't go hungry on the diet. But a lot of us eat for taste or boredom, not because we are hungry, and that is what you are trying to stop yourself doing.

4 Set goals

Set yourself small goals, little and often, and then reward yourself when you reach them. But not with food! If you decide you'll have a holiday or buy a new car if you lose six stone, that might be too far off to keep you motivated. Why not monitor your progress in pounds and have little rewards each time you hit the target? Perhaps you might get your partner to agree to take you out to the cinema or the theatre or a nightclub (but keep off the drink) every time you become another seven pounds lighter. Do whatever you can think of that will encourage *you* to keep on course.

5 Don't think thin

Think "happy weight" instead. I'm convinced that everyone has a weight at which they feel most comfortable and happy — although they may not have been there for so long that they have forgotten what it is. *Your* happy weight may be a fair bit heavier than what the models in magazines seem to be telling you to be happy at. So don't punish yourself by drooling over long leggy ultra-slim lovelies or svelte-looking males and telling yourself that you'll be like that next spring. Maybe you will and maybe you won't. If a weight is below what nature intended, you'll be suffering all kinds of self-deprivations to keep below your norm — and it isn't worth it or even a good idea. So don't think thin. Think healthy. You'll know when you've hit it, believe me.

6 Learn to think low-cal

There will be times when you have to come off the diet because you are away from home. (We'll be dealing with that in the next chapter.) But don't think that just because you can't stick to the rigid pattern you know, you might as well blow it for a day. That will be fatal. Re-educating your appetite means taking your new-found food-sense with you wherever you have to go. And it doesn't mean your poor old palate will be pleasure-starved forever. Lots of the tastiest meals are surprisingly low in calories. That is something that Myra discovered when she wanted to cook some special meals at home for guests. She even said she has found it a challenge to make meals that aren't fattening but fun.

Here are a few of Myra's specials to set you off thinking up your own ideas.

MYRA'S CHICKEN CASSEROLE (serves 4)

8 chicken portions	*bouquet garni*
8 oz onions	*clove of garlic*
8 oz carrots	*ground black pepper*
chopped celery	*2 chicken stock cubes*
1 tin tomatoes	

Skin the chicken joints and place in a casserole. Add chopped onions, carrots, celery, tomatoes, bouquet garni, garlic and black pepper. Mix the stock cubes with 1½ pints of water and add to casserole. Cook in a moderate oven (350°F, Mark 4) for one and a half hours or until tender. Serve with broccoli and steamed courgettes.

MYRA'S STUFFED AUBERGINES (serves 8)

2 lb lean minced beef	*dash of Worcester sauce*
8 oz chopped onions	*3 teaspoons Bovril*
clove of garlic	*black pepper*
mixed herbs	*8 aubergines*
½ pint tomato juice	*breadcrumbs*

Put minced beef in a heavy-based pan, cover with water and bring to the boil for five minutes. Pour off liquid, then add onions, crushed garlic, herbs and tomato juice. Mix Bovril and Worcester sauce with a little hot water and add to the mince. Simmer for 45 minutes or until tender.

Place aubergines in water and simmer until skins start to wrinkle (do not overcook). Cut in half and scoop out flesh and mix with minced beef. Fill the aubergine shells with the mixture and bake in a moderate oven for half an hour. Cover with very fine breadcrumbs and place under grill to brown.

MYRA'S SIMPLE STEAMED FISH (serves 4)

4 8 oz fillets of white fish	*lemon juice, black pepper*

Put the fish on a plate and season with black pepper and lemon juice. Cover with a lid. Place plate on top of pan of boiling water and cook until the fish has a milky texture. Serve with coleslaw salad or poached mushrooms.

MYRA'S COLESLAW SALAD

grated white cabbage	*½ teaspoon dry mustard*
grated onion	*2/3 tablespoons skimmed milk*
sliced onion	*black pepper*
sliced green pepper	*liquid sweetener*
sliced red pepper	*white wine vinegar*

Mix the vegetables together in a bowl, then dress with dry mustard mixed with 2 or 3 tablespoons of skimmed milk, black pepper and liquid sweetener. Emulsify with white wine vinegar until the dressing thickens.

Now, I was able to keep right out of the kitchen but Myra wasn't, and I admire the way that she stuck to her guns despite always *having* to think about food — whereas I could try to forget about it till a meal appeared on the table. That's why it is easier to feed the whole family along the lines of your diet.

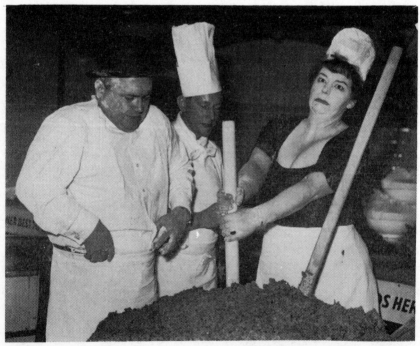

Making a 160 lb Christmas pudding (mostly Australian dried fruit!) in 1958

Temptation outside the house

When you are at home you can just about convince yourself that the world is full of cottage cheese and cucumber. It's once you get outside the safe zone that temptation really hits you. Steamed fish doesn't seem to appear on the menu in your run-of-the-mill lunchtime caff, I've discovered. But don't let that put you off. I've now had months of experience of picking my way between allowed and non-allowed portions in hotels and bars and restaurants across the world and I'm quite a dab hand at detecting fattening foods even when they are cleverly disguised by thin-sounding foreign names. Here's my tried and tested guide to sticking to the straight and ending up narrow.

Holidays
The first thing I had to learn to forget was the habit of drinking on the plane when travelling abroad. If it is a long flight it isn't a good idea to drink alcohol anyway — because if you and it are up in the air at the time, it tends to dehydrate you which just makes jetlag worse. I stick to mineral water, eat the salady parts only of the plastic lunch and try to sleep my way across several time zones.

It is very easy to get confused into eating more than your allotted share of meals a day if you started out in one country after lunch and arrived in the next one before breakfast the same day. My own trick is to keep my watch to English time throughout my holiday so that I can make sure I eat and drink at more or less the times I would have done in England. Nowadays I go straight to the hotel and sleep when I arrive to help me adjust to local time. (In the old days I used to adjust with a slap-up meal.)

Wherever you are, you have got to watch out for the vagaries of local cooking. A salad might seem slimming enough, but if you order it in Spain you're more likely to get a cold oil soup with bits of lettuce floating in it. The one phrase in Spanish I can now trip off my tongue is "sin aceite" — without oil. In fact, the one essential for the slimming holiday-maker's suitcase, besides the suntan cream and the anti-insect bite lotion, is a phrase book that lists all the likely local foods you'll get in restaurants. To be learnt by heart are words like "fried" and "roast potatoes" and "cream" so that you can bellow them out whilst making all the accompanying hand movements that signify "no". For instance, in Majorca — where Myra and I have a home — fish always tends to be fried, even if it doesn't say so on the menu.

One of the Spaniards' endearing but dangerous traits is to bring you "tapas" free with drinks in bars. These are delightful little snacks, ranging from stuffed olives to small chunks of bread sodden in fat and covered with a generous coil of bacon. If you have several drinks, you can actually have consumed the equivalent of a full meal before you leave to go to a restaurant for dinner. Try to get rid of your tapas discreetly — but not in the direction of your stomach. Often in Spanish bars there are children roaming about at all hours who would be delighted to gobble them up.

In Spain it hurts to turn down the red wine, so plentiful and cheap, but stick to your guns — and the mineral water. You won't find low-cal cokes or lemonade in the bars.

Wherever you are, unfortunately, you can't afford to sit back and relax when you have ordered what you think sounds an innocent dish. I remember Myra nearly throwing a fit when we chose barbecued steaks to eat while on holiday in Barbados. She suddenly saw our precious steaks being drenched in oil before they were put on the grill. Urgent semaphore signals ensued to save them.

The Greeks, in many restaurants, have the marvellous habit of inviting you into the kitchen to survey the delights of what they are offering for dinner. Either they are exceptionally proud of their prowess or else it saves on menus. Whatever the reason, it gives the figure-conscious fatty a quick chance to check what constitutes the sauces in which everything is swimming.

In Italy, need I say it, keep off the pasta. And watch what you get in France. The French love to cook with cream and butter so you'll really need your phrase book.

It isn't all quite as bad as it seems because there are still a lot of tasty goodies left on the menu that won't put paid to your diet with the very first bite. And everyone is always exceptionally keen to oblige.

Meanwhile, don't let the sun go to your head. When I'm lying on the beach these days, it is mineral water or soda with ice and lemon I drink for refreshers. Keep your eyes closed when they come round selling ices and sugary drinks, even though it is so much easier just to stretch out an arm than to weave through densely-packed sun-bronzed bodies and negotiate unexpected traps, like upturned buckets, to the nearest bar.

Some people, if they have dieted down to their desired weight and are simply trying to maintain it, choose to lose a bit extra before they set off for southern shores and so free themselves to indulge in a little of the local luxuries. I wouldn't dare tread that path myself. As a reformed fatty, I couldn't trust myself to chance my arm — particularly the one that reaches out towards plates.

Eating out at home
If you are dieting for life, like me, it doesn't mean that you can't go out and enjoy a good restaurant meal. It just means a mental weigh-in of what's on the menu.

Have a starter, as long as it is melon or fruit juice or half a grapefruit. Don't even let your eye linger over the antipasta and whitebait and avocado and egg mayonnaise.

White fish is always a good main course and if it does come with a sauce you can scrape it off but still be left with a little of the taste. If you go for roast chicken, don't eat the skin. Pass up everything in batter and breadcrumbs in favour of good guys like liver and kidneys. If you order a grill, check the meat won't be metamorphosed by fat or oil first.

Most restaurants swathe their vegetables in butter, so ask for them plain if you can. If in doubt, opt for an un-dressed salad.

And keep your eyes off the dessert trolley. If you can pass up dessert altogether, do. If not, it is down to sorbet or fresh fruit salad. If you stick to that rule, you need not even torment yourself with reading the names of the sweets that are on the menu. Just keep your eyes shut and order. Rare is the restaurant that doesn't offer fruit in some fairly innocent form.

If you have to drink, keep to whisky and mix it with three times as much water in your glass. It gives you the illusion you are one with the rest without the reality of paying for the privilege in poundage.

If you plan to precede your meal with a drink in the bar, don't ruin all before you start by dipping in the peanut dish. They might be little but they aren't any the less lethal for that.

Work-day lunches
Ah, the pitfalls of having to work late well into the lunch hour and then only having time to rush out and grab whatever is nearest to hand — usually a double decker egg mayonnaise sandwich or a sad-looking sausage roll that has been left in solitary state on the lunch bar counter. Resist, I urge you! If you can't make a point of getting out in time to seek for a salad, bring in something from home.

The loyal old lunch-box may be your lifeline if you've got a lot of travelling to do. Because isn't it always the way that just when the midday pangs come on, it is Sid's Transport Café that heaves into view, an oasis of bacon and thickly-buttered bread in an otherwise food-barren street?

Or else it's the late-night service station down the motorway where the salads are finished for the day and there is only an omelette on offer.

Parties
I'm not going to pretend it is fun being the only one at a party who is keeping his head when all around are happily losing theirs. Jokes never seem quite so funny when you're sober or is it just that the jokes get weaker as the liquor gets stronger? I find that my old ability to outdo the next man in army anecdotes that are outright invention is severely hampered by my new-found sobriety. Still, I also wake up the following morning without feeling as though I've being doing a turn in the tumble dryer, which is some small compensation at the time for the rigours of rectitude the night before.

I have now mastered the art of appearing to be drinking the hard stuff when in fact I'm stone-cold sober. I drink soda water laced with angostura bitters, the smell of which deceives even the heavy drinker. The drink that looks like a drink helps when dealing with those who feel you are flouting a lifetime's friendship if you don't join in the spirit of the thing. But the important part is to stay firm even in the face of the most importunate person. Pretend you belong to some obscure religious sect or that you're appearing in court tomorrow. Anything will do, because anything makes sense to someone who is half in his cups.

Whatever you do, *don't* feel guilty for not drinking. I can say, quite truthfully, that I have diabetes, but nowadays I don't even feel that I have to justify being on the wagon. People don't feel guilty for not smoking now, so why should we feel guilty for not drinking? It does just as much damage of a different kind and not only to one's waistline. "Everything in moderation" is my motto — especially when it comes to alcohol. Perhaps it will even stop me telling bad jokes ...

Exercise helps

Six months ago I thought of exercise as something I went through struggling to get out of an armchair. Walking upstairs was my equivalent of running the London marathon. Now I enjoy real exercise and see it as an essential adjunct to any diet. It isn't just good for you and all the things they say in keep-fit books. It actually helps your diet. Before you groan at the thought of regular exercise, run your eye down all the good news first.

Exercise beats boredom

If you are running around on a tennis court, swinging a golf club on a green or doing exercise to music at home, you'll be too busy to eat or think about eating. Keeping your arms active is one sure way to keep them out of the biscuit tin.

Exercise acts as a monitor

If you start off crawling round that tennis court rather than running, you'll know your diet is being successful when you have actually got the stomach-room to swing a backhand. It is all incentive to carry on with the diet.

Exercise aids circulation

Regular exercise does wonders for the blood. It can get round the body with less effort from your heart and lungs. So muscles, including the all-important heart muscle, receive more blood than before and can do more for you.

As the blood supply improves, the risks of heart disease start dropping. Lots of studies have shown that it is overweight people doing sedentary jobs who are likely to succumb to a heart attack. One survey looked at the spare-time exercise taken by 18,000 people in sit-down jobs, over a two year period. There was a definite link between exercise and fitness — and lack of heart disease.

Exercise makes you stronger

Whatever exercise you choose to do, whether it is swimming at the local baths or dancing at the Palais, there are benefits in other areas of your life. It won't finish you for the day when you walk upstairs and if you have to cross a room at speed to answer the telephone, you'll still have the energy left to speak, instead of pant, when you pick it up. Just twenty minutes exercise at least three times a week can be enough to start bringing your blood pressure and pulse rate down.

Exercise beats stress

Exercise is one safe way to deal with all the pent-up annoyances that accumulate throughout the day. When we have to deal with something stressful, our bodies get all geared up to cope — to fight or to flee. Blood starts pumping faster, adrenalin soars and all the systems not involved in the body defences slow down. Unfortunately our bodies are unable to tell the difference between being confronted with a raging bear in the front garden and having an argument with the boss. The bodily reaction is exactly the same but whereas it is put to use in the case of the bear — you'll run for your life — it has nothing to do but hang around causing tension in your body in the case of the boss (unless you make the questionable decision of slugging him in the jaw).

Getting rid of all that pent-up aggression in a non-violent

way, such as swinging a cricket bat or doing press-ups, does a lot to relax you both in body and mind. You will probably be able to sleep better at nights after it too.

Exercise improves your shape

Exercise licks you into shape in more ways than one. You'll find you have actually got a figure that isn't the identical twin of Humpty Dumpty. Not only that, but it will help improve your posture — and some women find it even helps their skin. What it all adds up to is a far happier self-image. You start to see that you look good, therefore you feel good. And when you feel good, you start to look even better still.

Exercise helps you to lose weight

If you have feverishly done your sums and come up with the conclusion that you would have to jog for about an hour to work off a few ounces of cheese, don't let it put you off. Exercise does help you lose weight and it isn't just a simple calorie-for-calorie exchange. Some people have lost nearly two stones in a year simply from incorporating a half hour's daily walk into their lifestyle, without dieting at all. The results are all the more dramatic if you do both together.

Stamina, strength and suppleness

The three direct effects of taking exercise are increases in your stamina, strength and suppleness. Stamina is what keeps you going, what gets you on to that disappearing bus before collapsing into a heap. Strength is all about muscle power, the ability to lift heavy weights — or even moderately heavy ones — without dropping them. Suppleness is the ability to move your body easily and therefore to move faster. It isn't something to dismiss as the province only of circus acrobats. If you don't do much exercise, your joints stiffen up, whatever age you are, and make even stretching or bending difficult.

Different sports provide different amounts of the three S's. If you want to concentrate on stamina, cycling, running, walking, swimming and even climbing stairs — all done vigorously — are the best. Golf and yoga and even housework won't do a lot for your staying power. They are effective for increasing your suppleness, however, as are dancing, gym, squash, keep-fit classes and swimming. Strength you'll get from digging the potato patch and from swimming — the only really all-round sport there is.

So don't think you have to become an up-at-dawn jogger round the park and into the cold shower person to get the benefits of exercise. It is even a myth that exercise first thing in the morning is the only time worth doing it. It doesn't matter when you exercise and it might even be wise to avoid early morning exertions as that is the time when your muscles are their most stiff and least cooperative.

Also, don't make the mistake of throwing yourself into a vigorous exercise routine, cycling and swimming and doing arm windmill exercises all over the place, if you have never left your armchair up till this moment. You can do yourself a lot of harm by overdoing it too fast. Check how fit your body is first. Can you walk up and down a flight of 15 steps without panting or being unable to speak at the end of it? If you can't, stop as soon as you get out of breath and go and see your doctor for his advice on how much exercise you should take and how often.

And don't, please don't, imagine that it is all right to jump in at the deep end and jog three miles a day just because you don't feel any immediate ill-effects after, apart from exhaustion. Bones that aren't used to exertion can crack if put to the test too soon. Women who have enthusiastically thrown themselves into keep-fit classes or dance sessions have been known to suffer hair-line cracks in the pelvis which they didn't notice at the time and which then got bigger.

Myra has suggested that I should perhaps join her keep-fit class or have press-up competitions by the side of the bed. I find that golf and walking are enough for me, but it is important to make the right decision for you. Whatever you do, whether solo or shared, it makes sense to enjoy it. So choose something that is a pleasure, not an endurance test. Suffering *isn't* the name of the game.

The benefits

If you are still with me this far, let me tell you of the joys that are to come.

I can cross my legs again. The last time I did that was back in the forties. I can also wear lace-up shoes again. It has been so long since I could bend down that far that I had to resort to slip-ons. I can even sing more lustily than before. And if you thought my singing was lusty enough, I can now hit a top "C" that would open the swing bridge at Warrington. I've just discovered my ears weren't meant to be part of my neck and actually sit on top of my shirt collar instead of in it.

I feel a bit like a sculptor now. What an amazing new skill, chipping away at a ton of lard and seeing an outline emerge from underneath it. When I was asked to pose for a photograph holding a 56 lb bag of potatoes, I could hardly even lift it. To think I once used to carry more than that weight every single place that I went.

I am so much more energetic, can breathe in lungfuls of fresh air without keeling over at the effort. I'm more confident, more alert — I wake up in the mornings now and know who I am. There isn't anything in my life that isn't easier to do without having to push a giant balloon in front of me. Nowadays I get through doors before my stomach.

Clothes are a newly discovered luxury. I'd forgotten what it was like being able to buy off the peg. In the old days the salesman would be shaking his head before I ever got up to the window. Now I swan about in up-to-date styles. I've given up trying to get all the old suits taken in — the pockets, once at the

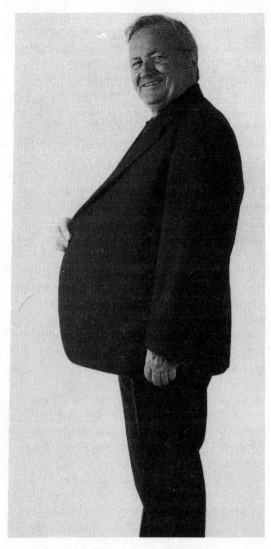

Photo David Secombe 1983

sides of my jackets, have all but disappeared under the bum flaps at the back.

It's nice to discover that there is room for me *and* the soap in the bath at the same time. And to find there is a space between me and my food-tray when I'm sitting on planes.

I even feel such a sense of triumph that it's a sort of self-righteous pleasure to walk into bars with Myra and say, "Gin and tonic for madame and a mineral water for me." (I'm getting to be a diet bore and I know it. But if people who've had enough resort to poking me in the ribs, at least now I have ribs to poke at.

I find I'm used by fat men's wives as a new line in nagging. "If that fat old Harry Secombe can do it, so can you," they say. And there is no answer to that because it is true. Which is why I have written this book.

I can honestly say, hand on heart — which is easier to reach now — that I haven't one real pang of regret for those puddings and pies and pastries and pancakes. It isn't just that life is so much more worth living. I'm all too aware that my bad old ways meant having no life left to live at all.

So it is over to you and I really do hope you will do it.

As for me, my only problem now is to come up with some thin-man jokes.